Body Alignment

Body Alignment

The creative person's guide
to balancing the material and the spiritual
to fulfil Life's Work and Purpose

Self Express
Publishing Division

Palmer, Monica S. (Monica Sylvia), 1959 -
Body Alignment: The creative person's guide to balancing the material and the spiritual to fulfil life's work and purpose

Includes bibliographical references.
ISBN 0-9683349-1-1

1. Mind and body. 2. New thought
3. Self-actualization(Psychology)
I. Title.

BF639.P34 1999 158.1 C99-931385-1

Published By:
Self Express
Box 428 STN. A
Toronto ON
M5W 1C2
Canada
tsheba@sympatico.ca

First Printing 1999

Maracle Press Limited

This work should not be relied upon for personal diagnosis or treatment, but used as a compliment to professional health care. Where there are major health concerns you must seek medical advice.

PART III - THE SEVEN PLANES OF HUMAN DEVELOPMENT

The eminent phrenologist, O. S. Fowler (1809-1887), wrote: "the faculties, are so embodied they act collectively, are the only instrumentalities of all we feel, do, and are; and collectively constitute our consciousness, selfhood, personality and life-entity"[1]. Therefore, a text on aligning body and spirit needs to take you, the reader, through an in-depth discovery, not only of the temperament and health of your own organism – although it is here the process must begin – but also of your spiritual self, your self-consciousness. In so doing, you will discover that there is no other purpose for the physical body other than that of the vehicle of the spirit.

Your sexuality is the key to achieving this alignment. Not as it is commonly used for of casual and hedonistic procreative acts, but for uniting man and woman in such a way that the exchange of the radiations of the soul engenders pure feeling and produces greater power for our highest achievements. Providing, of course, that the total involvement of sexual instinct remains subordinate to the creative-spiritual urge, expended for the fulfilment of your *life's work and purpose*, which alone paves the way to health, wealth and love.

To balance body (matter) and spirit, urge and feeling, vehicle and consciousness, this text allows you to reflect deeply on your spiritual well being, to eradicate all self-destructive tendencies and change attitudes. This spiritual shift, supported by correct nutrition, will change your blood-composition, which then alters DNA to fulfil *life's work and purpose*. This is what it means to govern the forces of nature.

This alignment, however, may, for some of us, require a major shift in attitude and desires – perhaps a radical 180 degree transformation – to regulate the excesses in life which have become propensities and now hold the spirit where it enjoys our dark and not-so-dark, inner sensations. In other words, your past self-destructive ways must die. You must "give yourself up".

With gladly "giving yourself up" comes an inner emptiness and the creative urge to fill it, that is, inner fulfilment. This approach alone guarantees the development of inner stability for that speedy and effortless clearing within the faculties for the expression of Supreme Divine Beauty in all your thoughts, intuitive perceptions and deeds.

Then will you come to understand that life is an actual investment for which strict inner balance yields compound interest, in the perfecting of your work – whatever it may be. You will learn that wealth is not determined by material possession but by your inner worth; only then will it serve you, instead of the other way around. You become that creative human being to whom everything you need for your happiness and well-being flows.

And as the Universe offers you everything of beauty that it contains, you will find that you can bear all your fortunes with only dignity and humility. You will also notice that there gradually arises within you the compulsion to extend a compassionate hand to assist others in fulfilling their creative endeavors, and to those still languishing in their darkness and despair. In this lies the fulfilment of the command: *Love thy neighbor as thyself.* For love is the fruit of volition.

The fundamental principle of Body Alignment rests upon the recognition that, "human being is a spirit". Spirit is the dominant power or force which transforms all that is Nature, human nature as well. It is the established position, therefore, that body alignment can only be achieved when one recognises that the spiritual governs, influences and moulds the material (the intellectual brain). With this, comes all tools necessary to realign the different energies of being.

But what do we know about spirit? There is the materialist dialectic that nature is fundamental to all that exists, that the spiritual is the product of the material. But in the creative ordinance of things this hypothesis is reversed. Nature, the spiritual effects of friction and amalgamation, is of three dimensions: (1) that which we can see with the physical eyes, (2) that which we can only sense or observe the effects of, and (3) that which perpetuates and multiplies all forms, be it another human life or other realities – world without end. Basically, nature is the world around us, or reality as it appears around us, and human nature is the way we affect this world.

Given that the world revolves around us, human beings are the dominant force in the centre of the Universe. Hence nature is not primary. It is the human spirit, which bears within itself an executive and preservative motivating force to create our realities with absolute consistency. That we exist is in the World of Gross Dense Matter, part of Nature, points also to the density of our conscious recognition, the result of the immutable Law of Gravitation where species of like consistencies cool off, group together and form worlds.

Nature – which consists of matter, that is, descending precipitation which, in the Law of Attraction of Homogenous Species, has cooled and settled in the slackening pressure of the rotation of Creation – is an ejection from a higher dominant species upon which it is dependent for its sustenance; not vice-versa. This force is the Primordial Source of All Things – including the Spiritual. So if spirit is not a product of Nature, we are not our material bodies, but are a lower species of this Primordial Form, the starting point of all things, in which lies unity and perfection.

And as with every sphere in Creation, movement begins with the lightest species above and, continuing downward, ends with the heaviest and densest. Spirit is the lighter, more fluid part of being – the Inner Voice – the urge we feel deep down, so pervious it penetrates the lower passions and desires and moulds even the gross physical body. Although separate form Nature, spirit remains its driving force.

This is what those who proudly calls themselves materialists find hard to grasp. Reality to them is only what they see – their activities and the fruit of their desires in the World of Matter. What can be validated they call science, anything else, empiric, quackery. For the most part, they allow their intellect, which is of matter, to absorb its stimulation from the visible world around and from thought-forms only, which it sends out remodeled again and again as its own reproduction and not from the spirit within. They cannot grasp that which is higher in nature, because being of the World of Matter their intellect is firmly bound to it. Their material brain allows everything to sink to its limit in accordance with the laws of its own nature and subjugates their spirit. Hence their inferior way of thinking.

Spirit lies beyond the boundaries of the intellect, separated by law due to the nature of its species. Hence the intellect cannot sojourn in the domain of spirit, much less make judgement upon it. Intellect merely serves to make movement possible in the most dense matter – to think, to see, to act. To live in the domain of thought is to live life in reverse, because this places the intellect above the spirit. It subjugates our innermost urges and estranges us from our spiritual nature, so much so that the very word "spirit" resonates within many of us with an unnerving, awkward feeling. We can longer see or hear anything spiritual, and any creative impulses or inspirations leading to the spirit is cut off as are our endeavors to fulfil our purpose in the field of activity.

Hence, to again understand spirit, so as to work with it, we must now painfully strive upwards from below; from that place where our superimposed intellect, with its limited capacity to comprehend, obstructs the broader transparency of our higher spiritual reality. Only within our inherent spiritual makeup can we stand in the middle of this gigantic mechanism called Nature, surrounded by activities that partly stream towards us and partly radiate from us. A constant intertwining, knotting, and loosening, building up and pulling down. Each change brings new realities, which is, maturity in our consciousness. A change in which today's reality becomes yesterday's error, which again may contain some grain of truth when looked back upon in the future. That does not mean, however, that reality itself changes, only the way we see it.

The sentient entity – spirit – which is highest of all metabolic activity and exists in unison with animistic (elemental) powers, forms the wonder-working machinery of the mind; creates all our functions, capacities and virtues; and forms things around us, including the physical body. Yet we waste precious time analysing the components of complicated machines and systems and other inanimate objects, or vegetal life, while the human spirit, which alone enjoys, suffers, lives forever, constitutes existence, and is the Creator's crowning work, does not receive supreme attention.

What Is Spirit

The closest we can come to truly understanding spirit and how it works in matter is to return to that period before birth, midway through pregnancy, the point of incarnation of spirit into the material body. This is when our embryonic or primordial germ cells began to differentiate from one another and from the individual organs of the body, for example, the heart, brain, liver, and lymphatic system, all based on "preprogrammed" genetic information. At this juncture, the astral prototype of what we will be and look like begins to form in organic conditions which indicate our character – be it good or evil; will we be healthy or sickly, thin or obese, tall or short, attractive or unattractive – or at least have a predisposition to any of the above. This is where parentage imparts *hereditary organic quality* – good or defected genes – along with life itself, heredity being the paramount condition and instrumentality. The predetermined stage of incarnation connects us with those parents and surroundings we are attracted to, and with which we share common backgrounds in the interpretation of reality and attitude towards life. Such stems from the adamantine law of homogeneity, and could not happen otherwise. Our chance at life depends mainly on the nature of our parents' souls, partly on their states of body and health; their mutual love or want of it; diet and lifestyle; and other like primal life-conditions and causes.

Here, at incarnation, invisible to the eyes or x-rays, are the spirit-components of the cells which give rise to the formation of elementary particles and atoms. These spirit-particles connect with the spiritual radiation of the human spirit incarnated in the physical body.

On the gross physical level, however, these atoms combine to form our cells' DNA (deoxyribonucleic acid) – the genetic synthesising factor which influences our behavior – and are compounded into protein-germs to form their main building block. The word protein comes form the Greek word, *proteios* or "primary"; proteins are large numbers of organic compounds that make up all living organisms and are essential to their function. Enzymes, hormones and antibodies are basically protein substances called substrates. These three major substrates, which rapidly combine with other substrates in the blood, catalyse the numerous, electrical, chemical and physical functions of the body.

Spiritual radiation contributes to the formation of human blood. This accounts not only for the difference between human blood and animal blood, but for the different formulae among human beings – O, A, B, and AB. If the material body alone formed the blood, there would be far greater similarity not only between humans and animals, but between every human being. The difference depends upon the spirit.

The atoms, with their primitive protein-germ compounds suitable for human cell development are collected by the soul wishing to incarnate from the parents concerned and the atmosphere. As with every life form, on reproducing, its species member passes on specific genetic instructions on how to intercept, transform, and release this spiritualised energy back into the environment during its life-span.

These atoms are shaped by the spirit to form its earthly body and held firmly together by a more pervious enzymatic-like substrate found, to a greater or lesser degree, in the bodies of all living things, the so-called mysterious Elixir of Life. So what is this substance drawn from the atmosphere around us, bearing atoms which continually change as we mature in consciousness? Where changes or paradigm shifts appear with new recognition of the journey to self-consciousness?

It is nothing other than ethereal substantiality, the soul's essence, the delicately active substrate of our desires or intuitive volition which brings life or movement to material form. This finer ethereal matter is our spiritualised or electrical impulse, that which the life-giving rays of the sun also contain and from which all living organisms derive their life-force. For this reason, the sun remains indispensable. No life-form would thrive without it – be it mineral, plant, animal or human.

This spiritual impulse is the condition for the true experiencing of the soul. Our deep desires, or rather, sincere volition (mere desiring or faint effort produced by weak volition cannot withstand the sudden tremendous ethereal pressure) forms the lever that releases spiritual power waves penetrating the entire Universe. The Universe always waits for this impulse to release spiritual power which we manifest in our works.

Boyle's law holds that the pressure of a given mass of gas is inversely proportional to its volume at a constant pressure. We can see why the release of spiritual power allows us to exert tremendous influence upon this world, which, at the same time, invest us with personal responsibility; for whoever brings form to perfection must take responsibility for the done deed – be it good or evil. The spiritual vigour behind each our thoughts determines the level of pressure and condensation which produces the quality of our activity – magnetic or repulsive, strong or weak – which in the end becomes our reality. Reality (the effect) is therefore proportional to inner power, importance and nature of our thoughts and perceptions. Hence the saying: Life is what you make it.

The soul remains our latent powerful energy source. From the soul level alone surfaces the impulses for our highest creative expressions or our self-destruction. The more spiritualised it is, the more powerful it becomes, and the greater is the ability to nurture our creative processes in form manifestations.

Researchers at the University of Manchester in northern England claim to have found the key to destroying resistant tumors in a protein enzyme called Bak, which triggers self-destruction in damaged cells. But they fail to understand why some 12 percent of the 52 million deaths around the globe in 1997 were due to cancer, in that most tumors resist chemotherapy and other drugs, and only a third of all cancer cases can be cured.

Until they realise that not only genetics but also spirit-radiation lies behind the forming of cells, all findings remain inconclusive. In fact, they will forever fail to see this spiritual activity behind the aligning and misaligning, tearing down and building up, living and dying of all matter (cells). Only then will they understand that cellular behavior is shaped by genes as well as by culture.

Their answer lies in proteolytic activity of cells. The spiritual component causes the chemical protein to behave like chameleon, changing its form and predisposition based on (1) the law of development and (2) our thoughts and wishes. The process shows itself more conspicuously at the onset of puberty.

Take the thymus for example. Divided internally by cross walls into many lobules, each full of T-lymphocytes (white blood cells associated with antibody production), it doubles its size by puberty. After that it gradually shrinks, its functional tissue replaced by fatty tissues. In infancy the thymus controls the development of lymphoid tissue and immune response to microbes and foreign proteins (accounting for allergic reactions, autoimmunity, and rejection of organ transplants). After puberty, we develop distinctive molecules that identify us as "self", different systems of cells coexisting in complete harmony with other organisms. The immune system is able to distinguish between "self", the biological self-protecting and self-healing forces of the organism, and "non-self", an antigen, and produces antibodies to attack any tissue or body fluid that does not carry a self-marker, for they are seen as invaders. This is the foundation of individuality.

Matured sperm cells do not appear until this stage of immune system development, which are then separated from the bloodstream. What effect, then, does puberty have on the proteolytic activity behind cell formation? Why is there no further demand on the thymus to continue its childhood function? Because puberty marks the time of conscious connection with the spiritual radiations pulsating downward through the Universe. We connect with them in various ways. *The resultant union of spirit and body (matter) forms a halo around the body giving it a special aura which protects and defends, and, at the same time, connects the soul with its wider environment.*

Visible biological changes is but the effect of the inner shaping the outer body form. The union and alliance of spirit and matter produce heat-emanations and radiations which cause cell to split, releasing hormones into the blood stream. The mysterious force behind this process is the awakening of generative power.

Generative Power

Generative power has long been associated with phallicism, the adoration of the phallus, the male organ of procreation and its counterpart organs of female fertility – both manifestations of gross nature worship. Generative power, however, concerns self-consciousness. We become conscious of our sexuality, that is, conscious of the direction in which we strive to develop the abilities – in the compelling and energetic masculine (positive) or the quiet, preserving feminine (negative) way – conscious of spiritual life. The urge for sexual intercourse is of secondary importance in this procreative process.

As soon as generative power sets in so does responsibility, the critical turning point in the life of every individual. While our thoughts, perceptions and actions must be governed to adhere to social laws of behavior, they also become the means to our immune protection and defense, *i.e.*, leukocyte reaction. Any stimulation upon the nervous system – emotional or mental – the hypothalamus directs protein-based endocrine hormones to form antibodies. Good and noble thoughts and desires bring health and well being. Dark or even not-so-dark thoughts and desires attract influences of similar nature which afflict the body with sickness and disease. In addition to attracting unhealthy environments, the hypothalamus also influences the body's drives towards the wrong nutrition, lifestyle and emotional behavior. This creates regulatory rigidity or restriction in the otherwise fluid flow of the substrate in the organism, psychologically as well as spiritually. Primitive "friendly" protein cell particles – which otherwise support the organism – begin to circulate in the blood, reproducing and generating infinite numbers of negative or "bad" bacteria and parasites of different shapes and forms to afflict its host, causing enzymatic reduction and oxygen deficiency.

A diet predominant in animal protein and fat increases the size of microorganisms as they develop into harmful bacteria while leukocyte mobility decreases. As we age, naturally there is a reduction of antibodies, our leukocyte reaction to infection wanes. The result is the numerous resistance-lowering factors such as metabolic, degenerative or consumptive and autoimmune diseases: rheumatism, arthritis, diabetes, gout, tumors of every type, anemia, leukemia, cerebral sclerosis, paralysis. This is a state wherein the immune system cannot distinguish unhealthy mesenchyme from "self", because viruses infect the antibody forming cell, so the body actually attacks itself.

Such afflictions Krebs quoted the scientists Pischinger and Keller as saying, is attributed to "mesenchymal block", otherwise termed regulatory blockage. The mesenchyme tissue is loosely organised and the individual cells migrate to different parts of the body where they form most of the skeletal and connective tissue, the blood and blood system, and the visceral (smooth) muscles, and perform such functions as maintaining osmotic pressure, optimal ion mixture and acid-base equilibrium by means of a continuous substance exchange between the blood and cells. According to Pischinger, he wrote, mesenchyme tissue "is the bearer of the undifferentiated and unconscious life function and state, of the holistic function in the organism and thus the basis of general and nonspecific resistance regulation"[2].

Dr. G. L. Freeman, however, took the observation further – to the physic level[3]. He noted that on this level the substrate may even become permanently fixated, especially when some persistent motivational excitant is thwarted from attaining an adequate discharge. Such postural fixation, he pointed out, explains the loss of contact with reality of many psychotic patients. This affirms that spirit is the greatest determinant of behavior, both external and internal (organic). When an individual in such a case firmly sets out on a specific course, the unconscious patterns dominate in a stereotypic way, leaving external influences (counselling, admonition) to have little effect. No amount of persuasion will change this individual's outlook on life.

Body Alignment through Change in Mental Attitude

Here, within the cell's nucleus – its personalised molecular structuring – the work of body alignment must begin through changes in our mental attitude and diet. Our faulty genetic disposition starts in the nucleus, which continuously influences our behavior – sexually and otherwise – as well as our beliefs, traumatising and misaligning our cells. This tension weakens spiritual radiation to the point that it is hardly able to influence the function of cells and organs, in order to achieve or maintain "radiant health".

When the refreshing and animating alternating spirit-current does not flow through the human system to continue the necessary "cycle of radiation"[4], a division is hewn between the ethereal (soul) and the material bodies (worlds), between the feminine (intuitive) and the masculine (intellectual) energies, and within the personality – the inner dichotomy. By the law of gravitation, the heavier, more gross species are bound to sink to the homogenous kind, to dominate. Hence the overstimulation to the sensual instincts and gravitation to the pleasures of this world.

Inadvertently, we shut out the good and noble influences that could mould our conscience, warn and nudge, though not force. When we lull our conscience to sleep by not heeding its warnings and nudges, at first it gives us no peace. This is a cry, the actual distress, of the conscience. To continue along our self-destructive path, is to divide the innermost self. Voluntarily we erect barriers between ourselves and the radiations of guidance and succor dispensed from the Cosmos. We cannot help but chain ourselves to our base desires, restricting our ability to surge to spiritual heights.

Consequently, we cannot help but evade our spiritual obligations, until gradually both body and soul (psyche) become diseased. This long-standing dichotomy – affected by childhood experiences – influences the autonomic nervous system and flaws our emotional development in such a way that by adulthood - with dissatisfaction in work, relationships and marriage - the enormous pressure exerted on the subconscious paralyses the intuitive mind and cuts off the higher spiritual self.

This leaves many of us living unsuspectingly in spiritual apathy, neutered in our own power to affect any change in our lives. Exhausted and fed-up, many of us unconsciously believe that nothing can change, for the experiences of life since childhood have been nothing but struggle and hardship, affecting our attitude toward society.

Hence our spiritual weakness, or bareness, due to a deprivation of spirit-currents from the cycle or radiation – the harmonious working of the masculine and the feminine principles in our lives. It is why egotism is the order of the day, in direct opposition to the spiritual. Our actions are laced with cunning, lust, distrust, envy, hatred, arrogance and conceit, though spiritual blindness prevents us from recognising it. We extol our own sagacity yet draw from the knowledge of others, which is devoid of life. What we call knowledge is not knowledge because we do not personally experience it, until it is established in our consciousness to mold character.

The partial or complete deprivation of the spirit-currents accounts for the terrible crises in our everyday lives. It not only affects those closest in our lives, but rebounds with destructive force upon our wider surroundings, the entire planet, affecting the collective human race. Due to the creative power dwelling in the ethereal part of our being, every *intuitively perceived* thought immediately takes on form corresponding to the context of the thought; always connected by a cord to us, the producer, it is drawn away by the power of attraction of the homogenous species in all that is ethereal (emotional), and driven through the Universe with the currents constantly through it.

As these currents move through the Universe, so they move through the human body, in that the latter is but a *prototype*; in this lies the *perfection* of Creation. Therefore, if the soul become afflicted, so does the body.

Herein lies the link between spiritualised ethereal matter of the soul (the creative substance forming the pattern of our every disposition) and the physical body with its genetic pre-disposition, both factors determining character. Hence an understanding the composition and activity of the human physiology cannot be gained with scales, scalpels, and test tubes, but with a clear, free, spirit. Neither can such observation be made with a constrained spirit or one hampered by prejudice.

Body Alignment through Change in Diet

Recognising our specific predisposition as an important source of diagnostic information to begin alignment, relies first on a change in diet. With the correct choice of nutrition – based on individual temperament – you will begin to harmonise the radiations of the physical body with the spirit, so as to fulfil your *life's work and purpose*. For as long as the body suffers from ill-health, the soul also suffers and continues its self-destructive path.

In that protein is the fundament of cells, reconditioning the body and mind using correct nutrients is the way back to harmonious functioning. Diet alone, however, will not do, but correct nutrients will support the body's own capabilities for regeneration, allowing genuine healing to begin. This in turn strengthens, weakens or displaces certain blood radiations, so that the favorable radiation leads and widens the range of capacity for adaptation and further spiritual development. Restoring and maintaining blood in the condition peculiar to our true spiritual nature is the prerequisite for a receptive body, through which alone our inner life can manifest.

Such fortification of body and soul is essential, not only to restore impaired health, normalise behavior, and balance personality, but also to cultivate an immunity capable of effective resistance to impingements upon mind and body – from inside and outside, *i.e.*, from our own self-destructive tendencies and our social, environmental and psychic influences.

When a change in radiation cannot unite body and soul, however, the result is mental ill-health and/or the development of degenerative (cancerous) cells results, leading to pre-mature death – the most horrible experience. For the spirit deprived of supporting radiations pulsating through the Universe weakens from ongoing emotional and bodily tension. Too weak to make connection, it cannot maintain and strengthen the physical body which can only happen in the fulfilment of our *life's work and purpose*.

Supported by the correct choice of nutrients, sexuality is key to altering our genetic consistency – DNA – by the perpetual moderation of excesses in life. It is estimated that 17 percent of our genes are "junk" genes, that is, bearing no genetic information. These are the cells we are targeting, to imprint our new genetic information bearing our new mental attitude and behavior. With the help of enzymes derived form raw, wholesome foods or in supplement form, these cells will self-replicate, down through to our offspring. And what else are the major excesses in life but the insatiable appetite for food and sex?

Hence the ability to "master our destiny" lies in our own hands. We allow spiritual radiation to influence the physical body through the blood – carrying antibodies, enzymes and hormones – to regain, fortify and maintain health. Accordingly, we raise the spirit's threshold to unfold its ultimate power in the development of our buried talents and abilities. Bear in mind, however, that any personal success will also greatly depend upon our innermost conditions, *i.e.*, karmic entanglements (the reciprocal effect of one's past and present actions), thought patterns, personal goals, social surroundings, inner strength, and much more. In other words, the level of our spiritual maturity.

PART ONE

THE FOUR CLOAKS OF THE SPIRIT

We wear four different species of cloaks to cover and protect our delicate spiritual core in order for us to become active in the World of Matter. The number four symbolises anything that has taken on form.

Keep in mind that spirit is our innermost core, our primeval substance and remains an independent consistency. It is, however, the dominant and controlling power upon animistic and ethereal power and the physical. Its quality has to do with our "deep inner feelings".

The animistic cloak, which connects to the nervous system, carries its own motive power in its core. It animates and steers our thoughts, wishes and desires – the influences of the spirit – to become our experiences corresponding to will. The ethereal (soul) is the creative soil, the womb in which these thoughts and wishes take on form. It exerts the germinating or formative pressure we sometimes feel almost immediately after our thoughts and wishes are generated. The astral body in the prototype of these thoughts and wishes projected upon the physical body and its immediate surroundings, brings experiences of happiness or sadness, health and well-being, sickness and disease, or some predisposition to one or another.

We must distinguish between spirit and soul. Sometimes soul is used in place of spirit, because it is customary and feels familiar. However, soul is spirit clothed in its delicate ethereal and animistic cloaks, effecting the fourth, fifth and sixth cloaks (planes) of the human spirit, as explained in Part III. When the spirit severs itself from the World of Matter, it leaves the physical and astral (shadow) bodies behind. The soul remains with only ethereal and animistic bodies in the so-called beyond. Soul ceases to exists when finally, the pure ennobled spirit sheds these cloaks and enters the Spiritual Realm. It crosses the Animistic Bridge, of which animals, bearing souls originate.

Why does the spirit need these cloaks? If we read the Creation Story according to Genesis as a spiritual and not an earthly account, we will understand that to descend into the World of Matter in the pursuit of knowledge, which was to be gained only through experiences that leads to ego-consciousness, the spirit-seed needed to protect its delicate core. So it covered itself with the finest material on each of the planes in its descent to the earth plane.

The World of Matter refers to two species of matter alien to each other – the more pervious Ethereal Matter we can only sense within, and Gross Dense Matter we can see with the physical eyes and with the aid of instruments. Matter refers to that which is used to create form or covering; the intellect of Fine Dense Matter covers the dense physical brain, the astral body of Medium Dense Matter covers the soul.

The spirit-seed cloaked itself in animistic substance to bridge the Spiritual Realm and the World of Matter. Possessing its own motive force, the animistic body enabled the spirit-seed to penetrate Ethereal Matter – the so-called Garden of Eden – and humans became living souls (Genesis 2:7). In an unconscious urge to ego-consciousness, the spirit-seeds became conscious enough (subconscious) to allow the ethereal cloak to form in the likeness of the image of God. Finally, when its ethereal body was strong enough, it was absorbed in the coarse physical body in an earthly incarnation, born flesh and blood.

The animistic cloak is the motive power or the higher nervous (psychological) activity of the faculties of the mind which gives rise to knowledge, wisdom and understanding. Connected with, or the higher form of, the nervous system, it is that substantiality which binds forms as it allows itself to be bound. In other words, it is the transitory body for incoming spiritual light waves or impressions with which it binds to produce thought and clothes to materialise in some form of action. As impressions come, the animistic body impels the senses to action by way of feeling – the signal that something is about to happen.

Animistic activity within the nerve impulses involves three phases:

1. The Emotional Phase: stimulation of the involuntary (sympathetic) nervous system (whether excited or inhibited), as picked up by the intuitive brain (cerebellum).
2. The Mental Phase: intercourse between the intellectual and intuitive brains, exciting the latter to produce thought-form, and its exteriorisation (going out) which influences the bodily (peripheral) nerves and produces sensations.
3. The Psychic Phase: creative intelligence, determined by the ability of the brain as a whole, to separate feeling and desire from logic (rightness) and reason to manifest thought-form as experience, from which one can learn – self-knowledge. This concerns the strength or quality of one's nervous system, that is, one's emotional stability. It does not speak so much to one's ability to attend to a great many things in quick succession, but how in performing the thing at hand, one, not just temporarily but with constancy and permanence, resists competing factors (external stimuli which allow the mind to wander or distract attention) and suppresses passions, so as to dwell patiently on one thing till it is done. All this is achieved through a directedness of thought and feeling – self-consciousness. Few can take a thought to this phase.

Of the psychic phase, one is said to govern the forces of Nature and not become enslaved, hence a "master of one's own destiny", only intercepting those external influences which are of the same nature as the peculiar emotions of the soul. Here one separates the doer from the worker (imitator); the visionary from the dreamer; the victor from the victim; the producer from the consumer; the master from the slave.

Thus the animistic body bears within itself the executive and preserving motivating power of creative intelligence – encompassing the great spheres of intellect and intuitive perceptions, of thought and soul essence. In the creative process of form, it first creates an impression within the ethereal body as emotions, depending on personality, which project pictures upon the conscious brain as thought-forms. What manifests or transforms and how, indicates one's level of intelligence. The animistic body is capable of producing either good or evil effects. It has no will of its own, it is neutral power driven by our volitional desire.

Depending on the object of one's desire, animistic substance animates the intellectual faculties, triggering feelings to produce experience. Hence the saying: he who feels it knows it. We learn from this experience, a process in which the knower and the knowledge become one. In other words, one fully and consciously participate in the development of the thought-concept from mere inspiration and materialise it from within one's being. This is how we develop intelligence.

Even though deficient intellect produces poor intelligence, scholastic achievement does not improve intelligence. Intelligence cannot be acquired by cramming the brain with subject matter, for intelligence does not lie in the *instrument* "brain" but in the *quality* of a person's brain, how one works with the animistic forces to balance thought and bring it into being, such as Moses' ability to part the Red Sea, which others attribute to supernatural, occult powers. Intelligence is bound up in the radiation of our blood based on the experience of the soul over the ages. We bring this quality with our hereditary endowment upon incarnation into that environment we choose for ourselves. How we make use of intellect determines our level of intelligence.

Hence, intelligence lies above and beyond, and carries far more potential than education and all its associations. No social background, no university training, no association or social conditioning can *make* us intelligent, in the same way that differently endowed human brains cannot be equalised. How we develop our intellect, through the fundamental disposition peculiar only to our nature, is left to our free will, which determines the object of our desires and goals. Our surroundings, however, can support and further our individual disposition. But this will take much *self-control*, which is the highest earthly attainment as it controls all others.

Animistic power penetrates the ethereal substance of the soul to shape our realities as it generates life in the physical body. Its forced movement activates and supplies warmth and movement to the gross material body as well as its brain via the nervous system. The permeability of the ethereal cloak (soul), which depends on how unencumbered the mind is of thoughts and mundane concerns, permits animistic radiations to easily penetrate and spread this new warmth (light intelligence) and consequent movement of the spirit. Its binding property facilitates the union between body and spirit, intellect and perception, to bring about self-conscious awakening through changing blood composition. The most profound effect of its working is in the awakening of generative power.

GENERATIVE POWERS

This stupendous union of spirit and matter in every human being marks the onset of puberty. It results in the gradual awakening of generative power, allowing access to the great reservoir of creative energy. Generative power – mind force – can now be directed to penetrate untapped human potential. At the same time, based on one's level of intelligence, it determines how well – if at all – the intellectual brain can be animated to control the body's rhythms and urges, *i.e.*, self-control.

This immeasurable natural instinct primarily helps the spirit unfold its full action in the material world. All creative expression would be impossible without generative power; for it is the bridge or means for animation and self-control due to the spiritual influence upon the intellectual faculties. Generative power warms and brightens the intellect, and the intellect reciprocally supplies the spirit with its full power, its warmth and vitality, manifested in the inexplicable charm of youth.

Puberty marks the cycle when the photoreceptive pineal gland, which by the seventh year of childhood is fully developed structurally, becomes animated and opens to receive spiritual radiations, *i.e.*, uniform Universal Laws or energies penetrating the entire nervous and endocrine systems. The astral and ethereal bodies along with the spirit-seed also become receptive. Up to this stage one remains a child, no more developed than highly evolved animals, only conscious (of its existence), but not self-conscious.

A big step lies between consciousness and human self-conscious; the latter involves the free and conscious will to decide, with full responsibility. Even human laws understand this critical turning point in the cycle of every human being and nation. It determines when a young person is declared of age, and has gradually been reduced from 21 to 18. Even now debates consider whether it should be lowered further and, when to consider one insane (morally ignorant with an infirm brain), in that a crime can only mean a disordered organisation of the brain, since the instincts of a healthy brain can only be good, hence only produce loving self-conscious actions.

Spiritually, as long as the human spirit leads nothing but a life conscious of its existence, it must retain the name of "spirit-germ", even if one grows to a hundred years old. Only with further development towards self-consciousness does it cease to be a human spirit-germ and become a *human spirit*.

The opportunity for this is given at puberty when the pineal gland releases the photoreceptive hormone melatonin into the bloodstream. This is orchestrated by the hypothalamus with its regulating chemical messengers or the body's vital drives and activities, such as eating, drinking, sleeping, temperature regulation, emotional behavior, and sexual activity.

The penetrating colour-radiations chanelled through the pineal gland develop the various bodily cloaks around the spirit – the animistic body, the ethereal, astral, as well as the physical. The observable biological changes upon the latter remain but the effects of an inner spiritual activity shaping the outer.

Though animals and plants bear these coloured radiations within themselves, in humans they only become active at the onset of puberty, the time of spiritual awakening. In this cycle youths become self-conscious, conscious of their perception of reality, of the effects of their sexuality based on the nature of their goals and pursuits. Only then are they able to learn how to make *conscious* use of these radiations through the intuitive perceptions. It is said, "we begin to show our true colours", the true nature of the soul.

Biorhythm

Scientists at Cornell University recently discovered that all systems of the body are run by genetic biological clocks ticking in synchronicity. They found that plants, insects, and animals have basically the same genes for regulating their biological clocks – built-in timers that tell the organism when each day begins and ends. These built-in genes produce protein-enzymes embedded with DNA and harbor changing and repairing properties. In humans, however, the study reveals that these clocks control changes in body temperature, blood pressure, mental alertness, and various other rhythms.

What else could bring about these involuntary actions within humans, which the interceptive impulses of the conscious brain – the master clock – merely sustain or restrain to determine their effectiveness? What is the impetus for any such activity to respond to the unconscious spirit's willing at the time of need and release hormones throughout the body, affecting all clinical functions? This is a natural spontaneous response which, when out of synch, these scientists were able to reset human biological clocks by shining intense light on the back of subjects' knees.

The researchers concluded that photoreceptive hormones sense light and signal to a clock, which in turn oscillates in a 24-hour cycle and controls other genes that establish rhythms (patterns) throughout the body. Separate studies also show that many blind people with no conscious perception of light have normal biological clocks.

How then do humans absorb light, if not from the dispensing spiritual colour-radiations of the Universe? And since there is more to life than we can see, from the onset of adolescence, the functioning of these clocks are spiritual-effects. On the level of the psyche, however, they signal how to cultivate self-control, how to control temperament.

The resultant union and alliance of spiritual-radiations with the physical body emit heat and radiation brought about by the motive animistic substance, which allows each individual to produce his or her own definite kind of radiation – according to the condition of the different bodies. The effect is the formed halo around the physical body. This is recognised and called the "Od" or emanations, which form our electromagnetic field.

This halo which gives each body-form a special aura, protects and defends, and bridges with the spirit to its wider environment. It also affects the inner environment participating in the development of the spirit in its coarsest sense.

The aura is our real immune and psychic protection. The quality of its radiating halo decides the strength of the vibration absorbed from the radiating system of the Universe to energise the mind-body complex in coming to self-consciousness. It also protects us from harmful influences upon body and mind.

By virtue of our specific temperament, we begin to collect these colour-radiations streaming through us and pass them on in concentrated form through our thoughts into action. The elemental forces or faculties of the body now become fully operational.

Depending on the plane of development on which we stand, the species of matter which predominates in the character and decides the composition of this emanation – mental (rigidity) or ethereal (spontaneity). In the law the species of matter most strongly represented is the energy that will naturally predominate. The dominant energy exerts the greatest influence upon the soul and our surroundings. The absorption of these radiations is reflected in the forming of our unique characteristics, appearing stronger or weaker according to the nature of our thoughts, perceptions and actions.

Every stone, every plant and every animal absorbs the wave-lengths of certain colour-radiations and reflects others from their own characteristics, which, according to the condition of the cloak or body of form, is entirely different. These colours surrounds us in manifold ways in nature: the green meadows and bluish-green forest, the blue sea and sky, and all the myriad colours of animals, flowers, fruits and gemstones, creating that balancing and healing effect.

Before generative power, the process is said to resemble that of a baby's. Through these colour-radiations the material cloaks absorb only what is needed to mature. When generative power sets in, the spirit stands fully equipped, ready to confront this magnificent realm of radiations of all other species or realities. The gates are thrown open and an immediate connection is established on all levels of the physiology.

By adolescence we are able to observe faults and weaknesses that remained dormant throughout childhood. Our spirit also encounters powerful radiations of this great Universe, mainly through linking with other species of radiations: colour-radiations of the different species of thoughts, perceptions and actions, of the billions of different human beings, not to mention the different ground and solar ones. The uninterrupted exchange of radiations with other human beings, *i.e.*, the capacity to observe how others behave, *etc.*, generates the movement for self-conscious recognition to distinguish one's own unique character, for the requisite balance between body and spirit.

Having been faithfully watched over by parents or guardians and given the tools for life by means of *adequate* education, this turning point marks that part of life's journey where adolescents become free and dependent upon self alone, if they are to become inwardly strong. It marks the time to begin building self-confidence, which cannot be earned by having adoring parents, financial security or mere talent.

Spiritually, all youths *should* now be allowed to do battle and face opposition so that in gaining victory they can progress. Even if this requires leaving home all together. When with the requisite exertion and diligence youths struggle toward personal goals, their independent spirit builds self-respect and self-confidence, because their achievement results from their own efforts. Then can they truly mature into responsible citizens.

The natural development of the body even indicates its time to leave parents' loving protection so as to undertake their own subsistence. This urge is in fulfilment of the Law of Equilibrium (Balance), which enables every individual body to move, the only way for humans to complete tasks in life. This law also holds and sustains *the entire world,* for only through the balance of equilibrium can stars and globes pursue their respective courses and maintain themselves.

In learning that life is not only about receiving (the passive), but is balanced with exertion (the active), the giving of one's self, youths learn to appreciate the delicate balance between in all things: male and female; cause and effect; giving and taking; day and night; light and darkness; inhalation and exhalation; rest and activity; food intake and waste elimination. With this they establish equanimity between their intellectual and intuitive brain which gives the body the physical strength through the medium of the animistic. Such youths can hardly lead a life of inner conflict.

This strong self-creating impetus is only afforded to this young adulthood cycle, well up to the fourth plane of development[5] of the cyclic age of twenty eight – the end of the melancholic cycle. It declines steadily when adulthood – the choleric cycle – begins, the time when the apprenticeship cycle should give way to the manifestation of ingenuity and brilliance in our work. Neglect to make use of the generative powers in this earlier period to cast off our weaknesses and defects of character through self-conscious actions, is bound to show up as omissions, *i.e.*, failures, if, as adolescents, we had not already fallen through the cracks.

Hence puberty is the time to begin acting responsibly in order to maintain harmony of organic functions and a keen mind. This requires healthy blood-radiation. But for this to happen at the proper time, we must change the pattern of our thoughts and perceptions, mainly through the choice of diet and a complimentary lifestyle.

But instead of learning self-control, this strong motive mind-force is usually diverted to bring about destructive effects upon youths and their environment. Such rests in premature sexual indulgences, often resulting in unprepared and irresponsible parenting; stimulating the desire for sex be it in masturbating, reading or viewing of promiscuous material and being in bad company; or purely athletic ambitions with no energy left to serve true humanity. The mind is further aggravated with junk foods; smoking, stimulants and substance abuse, excessive drinking in student fraternities; the deprivation of sleep in the false mode of living. Even the compulsive reading of novels, occult and wrong psychic exercises forces the brain to appropriate this power of the mature body, only to dissipate it into these false and unnecessary activities – gradually weakening the mind and body.

Without the right complimentary moral education, youth will not realise that the awakening of generative powers means to develop what it takes to stand firmly in this world and influence it effectively, and at the same time receive protection to arm themselves against all wrong influences. They must realise that it is demanded of them to stand responsibly in Creation. Youth must recognise that generative power provides the opportunity to decide what is good and evil, giving them the urge to free themselves from internal or external influences that bind or seek to bind the spirit through the consequences of their desires.

Abd-ru-shin[6] describes generative power as *"the finest and noblest flower of all gross matter,* the highest the Gross Material Creation has to offer ... the pulsating life of the World of Matter, and it alone can form the bridge to Animistic Substantiality [elemental or intellectual faculties], which in turn acts as intermediary to the World of Spiritual substantiality [the expressions of the gifts and abilities]."

In the human faculties generative power is:

FIRE the intensity of creative impulse within the unbounded domain of Creative Intelligence engulfing the spirit and granting it cognition for the necessary observation of personal recognition.

WATER will power radiating its effect into all the worlds and sinking with irresistible force upon millions of smaller personalities, to dominate and bring about the fulfillment of wishes.

AIR the pressure produced from the resistance of the downward dispensing radiations of the Universe upon our upward volition of the soul; the main lever of human evolution which sets in motion the greatness of our innermost power for the development of our creative self, for it presses out everything we express, in words and deeds.

EARTH the intellectual ability to execute the high art of judgment for our defense and keen thinking, which surges like spears to achieve our highest good.

Generative Power and Sexual Instinct

Generative power, as already stated, has long been associated with phallicism, the adoration of the phallus, or male organ of procreation. But it's penetrative power upon the soul is what needs to be studied and adored. The consequent union from the physical urge to procreate, though vital, remains of secondary importance.

As the body matures, animistic substance permeating *primitive* germ cells, which before remained inactive in the gonads, undergo cell division and secrete hormones which stimulate the nerves and cause the body to "come on heat", or to be "set aglow". The endocrine glands which are particularly concerned with blood-radiation pass these hormones into the bloodstream. Subsequently, we become conscious of our sexual emanations, which unite male (positive) and female (negative), to act upon each other.

This metabolic reaction, however, is for the necessary stimulation and possible renewal of cells – procreation. This is the means by which cells of an organism transform energy, maintain their identity, and reproduce. This is the primary purpose of this exchange in sexual radiations which nature demands of all living species. It is how every mobile species in the World of Matter seek renewal and preservation.

However, generative instinct is independent of sexual instinct, otherwise called having nature. Nature has nothing to do with the spirit, in that spirit is not nature nor part of it; in the same way nature is not a part of spirit. One's body may mature sexually but the spirit may never direct generative energy to creative use, only downward to the procreative organs to act in an animal fashion.

Coitus, however, should serve only as an act of celebration of the joyous activity stemming from union; which can bring about spiritual consequences, *i.e.*, apart from the incarnation of another soul, help in our inner development. Sexual intercourse ensures the equally valuable and necessary process of an intimate fusion and mutual exchange of vibrations for two are striving to develop spiritual gifts, producing greater power for all their activities.

If adolescent education incorporates such knowledge from early teenage years, youth will understand that sex is not love. True love comes when they forge meaningful relationships before engaging in sexual acts. They will understand that love is a principle to create with, not to forge unions to guarantee sexual pleasure, social status, nor yielding to comfort and a life free from care. It should engender the desire for union where the male and female work actively and passively side by side, constantly striving towards one another for a common spiritual goal. A joint working together whereby the two can only achieve something which is perfect.

They must learn that intimate unions should be formed only where one finds the other partner stronger in those abilities he or she has undeveloped but needs as a compliment to fulfil both their creative ideals. In this alone lies the meaning, "destined for each other". In other words, each was born with the necessary psychic qualities to compliment the other. The two therefore become a full compliment, a united working of all the creative abilities of the spirit – positive and negative.

Generative power then serves to lift them, or rather, bring their activities to blossom and bear fruit. Joyfully and voluntarily they serve each other, and both toward spiritual ennoblement. Shoulder to shoulder and with a smile they face life's challenges and obstacles.

This achievement, however, sometimes requires developing the so-called Destructive Emotional Faculty, that is, in addition to being the lover makes one the exterminator as well. For the greater part of love is severity; a necessity for the progressive development of all that is formed. Love is a process which demands that everything formed is maintained and kept in perpetual motion, with the strictest consistency. We could therefore call love a quality control measure, by which anything not up to standard is expelled. A measure in which no weaknesses, illogical or sensual indulgence is found.

This means that at times we have to destroy anything that impedes our personal growth; cause pain to anyone who stands in the path of our happiness, for sometimes this is the only way others may come to understand themselves. This is justice, the other side of love. To over-cultivate the destructive emotion, however, is to pervert it toward violence; revenge; malice; even the disposition to murder.

On the other hand, youths should learn to tolerate those who are different from themselves and who make mistakes they consider below them. For as long as a person bears a normal brain, that is, is not over-cultivated or bearing a genetic deficiency, even with poor or moderate intelligence one can produce a useful intellect in some form or another and develop it into good intelligence.

Puberty is that time to direct generative power to liberate oneself in the striving to develop our natural talents and abilities, thus cultivating the mind. This prevents one from becoming the "one-talent individual" who buries other talents and embraces a life of poverty and covetousness, blaming others but self for misfortune.

Incompatible Unions

"Fatal attraction", or destructive relationships happen when a union, whether for mere companionship or intimacy is forged with another who is unequal; that is, where there are no complimentary values or life-skills. Wherever two who are unequal are linked, the Law (of Gravity) ordains that the higher one is *pulled down*, because the lower one can never ascend beyond their level of conscious awareness.

This Primeval Law of Creation, thought it allows for all that is spiritual to ascend, also causes a higher spiritual one to descend, to retrogress to lower stages when two who are unequally yoked strive together. For no human spirit can raise the spirit of another even one step above the place as determined by its level of consciousness, no matter how highly evolved. It is easier for the higher spirit to descend.

In a voluntary and close union between two human spirits unequal in their maturity, the higher one *must* either descend or have its growth slowed by the other, who remains backward in his or her maturity and hangs upon the other like a weight through this tie. The same applies to forming peer groups. Hardly anyone possesses the inner strength to lead the less mature one in such a way that the other comes to his or her level. Youths should be informed of this from the earliest years. Not to give consideration to these things before they engage in relationships – business, social, personal or otherwise – will teach them that a complete severance from such unions is not so easy at all.

Thus it is sung: "Breaking up is so very hard to do". Because in their helplessness, the weaker soul hangs on to the stronger by a thread, much the same as a parasite to a luscious plant. The weaker soul can become very abusive, choke its support to death, in a fight for its sustenance, while the supporter feels guilty to eradicate this "thorn in its flesh" out of pity it may suffer or die.

This is what creates some of the most compelling dramas in our lives and, although painful, we cling to these feelings of negative emotions, which feed our enfeebled "ego". They result from deep-seated responses which surface out of our subconscious beliefs in servile love from our conditioning, culminated with our weaknesses and inadequacies. In these weaknesses we not only harm ourselves, but those we imagine we are pleasing. With this mentality we go through life giving everyone power over ourselves which keeps us down, be it the priest, educator, politician, family member, or anyone who plays upon our weak emotions.

Generative Power and Ageing

Generative power has no age-limit. It still exists even after sexual instinct has ceased whether by old-age or other factors. And so does melatonin, although its levels in the body decline with age. This has lead to the speculation that melatonin acts as an anti-aging hormone and is the subject of sensational claims that link it with enhanced sexual performance and the prevention of serious diseases such as Acquired Immune Deficiency Syndrome (AIDS), Alzheimer's disease, Parkinson's disease, arthritis, epilepsy, and hypertension. This has increased demand for this over-the-counter synthetic supplement which can have little effect if any.

According to Dr. Harald Krebs in: '*Humans & the Ageing Process:* "Ageing is a gradual process of change and transformation in the course of our lives. But again also means that, sooner or later in one's life, there comes a time when the regulatory mechanisms of bodily functions no longer coordinate with each other optimally, thus upsetting homeostasis. When ageing begins, the organism's adaptive ability changes, *i.e.*, adaptive mechanisms lose functionality partially or totally—but, at the same time, new adaptive mechanisms are developed or take on new quality."

It follows therefore that although many old-age dysfunctions are inevitable, most bodily afflictions can be prevented or at least slowed through direct mastery over the regulatory mechanisms of bodily functions by the human spirit early in life. The body which does not swing in rhythm with the spiritual-creative self cannot be maintained and strengthened through its work, but becomes aged and stressed, because it does not receive the spiritual nourishment it needs through the powerful currents of the mind.

This requires honoring the physical body as the temple for the spirit. Respect and preserve it as something inviolable, if it is to have any value at all. We must master our bodily implement and its urges and not become its slave. Chaining ourselves to our passions – over-cultivation of the intellect purely for academic excellence, over-indulgence in food and drink, the insatiable desire for sex and personal comfort – we direct generative instinct downward into the sheer pleasure of the brute, which only enfeebles the spirit and deprives it of the great impetus it so urgently needs to strive upwards.

In so doing, we suppress our conscience which nudge us always to do the right thing. Even when it is lulled to sleep in order to continue satisfying our selfish ambitions, it still gives us no peace. Finally, when suppressed altogether, a duality establishes within ourselves as erected barriers between us and our spiritual guidance which cuts off the latter, sometimes altogether. Without vigilantly striving to restore this relationship, before our adaptive mechanism loses its functionality, we will not be shown how to correctly widen our range of adaptability. This can only lead to errors, thus old-age afflictions – within the body and soul.

The ethereal cloak consists of three layers, or rather, three planes of development – Coarse, Medium and Fine Ethereal Matter. These are the fourth, fifth and sixth planes in the seven planes of human development, discussed in Part Three. For now it is enough to know that the fourth plane forms an intuitive bridge to the conscious brain; whereas the sixth plane is bridged with the seventh (the Spiritual Plane) by the Animistic Plane. The higher the development on each of these planes, the more fluid our thoughts and perceptions and the more we experience those momentary out-of-body transcendental and blissful experiences of the soul through activity. One with a developed ethereal cloak experiences life from what is called, "beyond time and space" that is, beyond that which the conscious brain is able to grasp.

The radiations of the fourth plane of Coarse Ethereal Matter in union with third plane of Fine Dense Matter, form the transitory point in the brain. Transitory in that the two different species of radiations can only unite (not fuse), because, subject to the law of form, two different species can only merge. Chemistry alerts us to the fact that the difference in species can even create insurmountable barriers.

Merging in this case permits two different kinds of forms and composition to develop from the radiations of the original species of matter, the effects of which remain within the range of the basic substance as determined by its origin. The resultant form is the human temperament[7] – the specific patterns of nervous response to internal and external stimuli, part genetically inherited and the other, of the nature of the individual's soul. The human temperament, though personal, remains material, because it is formed from the radiation of the of two different species of matter, not the spiritual. We could say it is etherised.

All stimuli upon the central nervous system produce a resistance at the transitory point in the brain which creates pressure and causes the blood to radiate. The pressure of resistance presses out all that we express, verbally or bodily, everything we manifest at any given time. And this radiation accords with the pattern of one's temperament, bodily instinct and feeling. It is different in each person – stronger or weaker according to the nature of one's volition and work, constituting different perceptions and feelings among individuals.

Hence the ethereal body, that brings life to the form of our thoughts and intuitive perceptions as willed by the spirit. This pervious cloak, of the nature of rich, moist soil prepared for sowing seedlings, anchors our thoughts and wishes until they develop and ripen at harvest, yielding many times over based on the intensity of volition.

It is here the dreaded and incisive activity of karma comes into effect; for this ethereal soil also has a rebounding effect. Sooner or later, upon maturity, everything we conceive in thoughts and wishes is bound to return to us. The stronger the urge, the greater the chance for development, be they good or evil desires. Thus it is said: "as we sow to the wind we reap the whirl wind".

If we continuously create wrong thoughts and actions, the reciprocal effect binds us by influencing our free will and giving it a pattern that can be estimated in advance. This is called stereotypical behavior. After some time one finds oneself unable to ever do the right thing, becoming not only a danger to oneself, but to society as well.

We can feel the ethereal body in that we feel the after-effects of everything we will within our beings. We can sense them, whether they be joy, exultation, sorrow, hatred or lust, even though we cannot touch them. As soon as the will gets to work, the force creates pressure. This pressure we feel within us as the urge rises to impregnate the ethereal body, also called the womb, before it rises to become a thought.

The pressure indicates that the ethereal body is substantial and active. Where there is no pressure there is no activity, no sensing. The fact that we feel pressure means something solid of the same substance is active, resulting in the pictures or impressions and the subsequent conceptions we form. We cannot perceive pictures or ideas from nothing. This very conception would mark the greatest gap in the laws of exact science. Something must be there, and something is there.

Every generative thought immediately creates in the Ethereal World corresponding forms, the density and vitality of which depend on the intuitive power of the generative thought concerned. Therefore what is called our "inner life" is that which produces a corresponding and similarly formed environment around us in the protective aura sheet. Our inner life attracts to us the circumstances of our desires whether it be people of like mind, a solution or guidance, chaos or suffering – all depending on the kind of seeds we have sown in the perception.

A recent study at the Hopital de la Salpetrière, Paris, headed by Dr. Varela and colleagues, identified this flow-pattern in the so called "crackle of activity" in the brain, the instant an impression is recognised, in this case a face. They noticed how, upon receiving a transmission, the brain blends the flood of information from the nerve sensors (senses) into an overall thought, the "binding problem". This led these neuroscientists to believe they had discovered to the key to consciousness.

They learned while monitoring the activity of the brain that, as their subjects studied ambiguous stimuli that looked meaningless, *i.e.*, pictures upside down in relation to pictures turned the right side up, in the latter, the brain actually binds different flows of information into a thought when assemblies of nerve cells synchronise, firing together with millisecond precision. They hypothesised that synchronisation in widely separated regions of the brain occurs only when the picture (impression) could be recognised as a face, corresponding to the moment of perception.

During these "gamma oscillations" – in a band of frequencies around 40 beats per second – nerve cells scattered across the brain synchronise to form a coherent group, much the same as millions of tiny lightbulbs switching on and off simultaneously. The scientists deduced that these waves of synchronised switching are the mechanism that transforms disparate activity in the brain into a conscious thought.

The study further revealed that the recognition of a picture was followed by action, in this case, the subjects responded by pushing a key. Thereafter, the firing neurons de-synchronised before another movement of brain waves entered into a new pattern of synchronicity. The peak of one wave always corresponded to face perception, and the next to the subject responding. The separation between the peaks, and thus of each thought, marks the "frame of time for cognitive life". This shifting from one cognitive state to the other has Dr. Verela perceiving that "there has to be a complete decrease in synchronicity, an active 'unglueing' of the brain patterns before the next thought can come up".

The study focused on pictures alone, but every longing, every prayer, every desire, good or evil, arises as an emotion and creates pressure in the brain which presses out our individual pattern of blood-radiation of temperamental behavior, stronger or weaker according to the nature and strength of the volition. Hence the different activity of feeling and perception, which leads to our actions. The predominant pattern of response to these emotions is identified as one's predominant temperament; that action which can be estimated in advance in the personality.

INTUITIVE PERCEPTION

To understand how the ethereal body works is to understand the nature of the intuitive perceptive brain, the Inner Voice. The human spirit expresses itself not through the intellectual brain, but solely through intuitive perception of the back brain (cerebellum), through its ganglion of nerve paths leading from the solar plexus. The intuitive brain is the main bridge between fluid spirit and the dense material world; between those Luminous Heights of Spirit (of lofty virtues) and the Darkness (carnal passions).

Only through intuitive perception can the pure Life from the Source of Light pulsate downward in the deepest gross material, and from here upwards again in the most glorious reciprocal action.

With pure intuitive perception we link these two worlds – the material and the spiritual – in one body. That is what makes human beings so unique, for only humans, due to the nature of our being are constituted in this way. Therefore, the Darkness (of matter) and the Light (of spirit) both form human character. Hence Light and Darkness are therefore possible in our every act.

Our actions are capable of bringing about both good and evil effects. Although the Darkness lurks about our consciousness, the bridge of intuitive perception forms that harmonious intercourse between the intellectual brain and the Planes of Ethereal Light, which alone brings understanding, *i.e.*, freedom from the Darkness (ignorance) by transforming the mind into its sheer brilliance – like that of twilight.

Today we have advocates of the wrong principles of the Darkness who, with their psycho-analysis and judicial powers, seek only to destroy those who with little self-reliance depend upon their counsel. We hear so much about "freedom of expression". Its meaning, however, lies not in guiding the people with the right knowledge founded upon Natural Laws, that may allow them to come to recognise their self-made inner conflicts and work to liberate themselves. It is based upon the wrong principle of "letting oneself go".

This allows for a social climate where there is no longer any privacy in our personal affairs and rights as we now see in sexual life and similar things. We see the majority of society has lost the feeling of shame which is an integral part of personal self-consciousness, a part of personality, and without which there is nothing individual. Voluntarily stripping themselves of their individuality, such denuded ones becomes so cosy in their affairs they see no need to cover up.

Those who would demand it otherwise, however, are forced to accept the systematic intrusion of this unnatural trend in that area of our lives they hold most private, in the form of constitutional laws enacted by the very ones chosen to lead our affairs in government. Sex rights no longer represents the right to make personal choices as long as such proclivities remain private affairs, it is a lifestyle forced upon society as acceptable with a stroke of the pen to pander to the electorate or appear liberal. Just imagine, pornographic rights and the right for women to go topless in public.

Such practices and perceptions let loose today, upon those who are weak-willed or too young to perceive right from wrong, is frightening. Still more pitiable is the quest for self-realisation in which one finds oneself controlled by the thoughts of others. It is as if their clothes are systematically torn off and new clothing forced upon them.

But when unnatural sexual proclivities are accepted as part of the "status quo", this is no longer about private choice. It speaks to a perversion of an entire society. What separates humans from animal is self-control, the restraint of the lower passions. Hence the more intense the feeling of shame, the nobler the sexual instinct and the higher the individual ranks spiritually. One's inner worth is measured by the greater or lesser degree of physical shame, which alone precludes all possibility of perversion.

Shame is the precious jewel which is an infallible standard and easily recognised. When we forcibly and wilfully push it aside under the guise of human rights, we encourage bestial behavior. Society retrogresses to an animal-man state, even below the level of animals. The same society resorts to barbarity measures in applying severe penalties without rehabilitation for the sex crimes of those swayed merely by impulse, those who do not have sufficient moral sense of restraint, which only makes them worse.

When the feeling of shame is choked and eradicated, the soul's finer and quite different feeling of shame will be simultaneously choked and the inner self consequently debased. Only the worst abject terror can ever reawaken this feeling of shame and end such a trend.

Sexual behavior is not the only concern here. This debasement occurs under the guise of progress: sports, festive celebrations, hygiene, fashion, children's education and other pretenses. Only when we set out to be "natural", *i.e.*, to listen attentively to our inner voice can we not disregard its warnings.

The Forming of Intuitive Perception

Intuitive perception is created with the strong power of spirit, through the emotions of the astral body (plane). The act of willing causes a particular emotion to radiate, immediately forming what is called a "picture without words". Every urge or generated thought creates a corresponding form upon the ethereal body, the density and vitality depending on the intuitive power of the generative thought concerned.

As the urge rises, an impression is made upon the frontal brain. Based on the nature of the various impressions received, the receiving intuitive back-brain, like a photographic plate, forms a picture of what is willed by the spirit or created by the strong power of intuitive volition. The intellectual brain takes over this picture as thoughts, remodels, condenses it into visible form - in the field of relativity. By so doing, it compresses the original perception into still narrower form, restrains it, and puts it more firmly together.

The final stage of this transmission through the frontal brain is the spoken word. The brain coins the thought anew and endeavors to describe it in words by issuing thoughts of similar nature so as to express it in language to fulfil a definite aim. The intellect forms words and sentences, which are but ethereal sound waves, producing new effects by the movement of these waves as they penetrate the speech organ. The intellectual brain can also directs the course of effect towards the organs of locomotion instead of speech, whereby words are replaced with writing or action.

THE ANDROGYNOUS (ETHEREAL) BODY

The intuitive brain is the so-called small or back brain. This designation, however, seems quite correct; for it captures the lesser role the feminine plays in today's patriarchal world. This portion of the brain serves as the negative reception of the higher spiritual impressions or influences coming in through the Cosmos. It is of the feminine nature to receive. The intellectual frontal brain on the other hand serves at the aerial that holds on to what comes into contact with it from the intuitive brain. Its masculine nature is to activate, to transform what has been received.

This is as far as it goes when it is said we bear both the masculine and the feminine working within ourselves. It does not speak to a bi-section or bi-sexuality, but the harmonious working of the two brains. The intellectual brain expressing in the field of objectivity and action; while the intuitive brain receiving impressions for the intellect to act upon.

For this reason the man, endowed with the gift of action, was built to perform the coarser, more mental, difficult and heavier tasks. In fact, for this reason his body is solidly designed. "Traditional" females (not modern woman) is found in the more nurturing domain, caring for and preserving life in general.

Good women falling for "bad boys" is perceived a social ill. But this becomes a problem only when the so-called good women are merely sexually attracted to these bad boys and not working from a higher moral place. In the natural ordinance of things, what these women are intuitively attracted to, is the originality, power, firmness, courage, passion, *etc.*, in the man. They love these qualities and dislikes the converse. The genuine man loves purity, exquisiteness, affection, maternal love, piety, taste, prudence, *etc.*, in woman and is repelled by the converse.

We could say this natural attraction is a built-in unconscious knowing of the Creative Principle, going back to the beginning of time. The principle which created man and woman with these complimentary values, even though the different Creation Stories of the different races and peoples are interpreted otherwise. Today woman fights for this equality and challenges the notion that she was created from the ribs of the man who, due to failure to perceive the truth about himself, appoints himself as her superior.

Such discourses will remain conflicting if we consider things figuratively, that is, from a masculine left brain's obstructed view and not from an ethereal point of view. Man, or rather, primeval man speaks to the androgynous (both male and female in one) spirit-seed. The separation of man and woman – the taking of the rib from the man – was an ethereal happening, in "the beyond". The deep sleep Adam fell into was the end of his first earth-life, to be reincarnated as man and Eve as woman.

The understanding behind the Creation Story according to Genesis is, that: for Adam (the first human-species) to survive on his own in the rough elements, the rougher, sterner, intuitive perceptions became dominant and was subsequently ejected to the dense material stronger man, separated from the delicate female part of being. In the lawful happening the coarser spiritual-masculine, the positive executing part, naturally must be ejected first. Because it is always the first to express, the active masculine was the first to sever itself from the spiritual substantiate so that the passive spiritual-feminine could remain separate. Pictorially we can say: both man and woman came into existence at the same time; the spiritual feminine came into existence when the coarser masculine severs itself ethereally.

This is why man and woman on earth, split species of the other, strive to travel life's path together. We constantly seek that soul mate, wherever he or she may be, for the restoration of the Unified Self. The Animistic supports this coming together spiritually by creating the sexual instinct in the material body; the desire preserves this union.

Distorted Soul (Sexuality)

Where there is a distortion at the soul level regarding the prescribed activity of original sex, the original form must also change, at least energetically. The spiritual, animistic and ethereal form of the body changes as soon as the spirit-germ alters its activity. If it changes from a negative to a predominantly positive activity, the female form must change into a male one, and vice versa, for the predominant nature of the activity shapes the form. Hence we find male souls born in female bodies and *vice-versa.*

Such possibility toward sexual distortion, however, was foreign to primeval man and woman. Primitive man was always in touch with his feminine side, he was never without love nor suppressed his emotions, but was never weak and yielding. Neither did the woman fail to support him or nurture his creation. Primeval human beings were too open to life and its co-operation with the higher ethereal spheres and were therefore incapable of anything unnatural. And it is this primitive behavior the so-called good woman still admires in the "bad boy".

THE FEMININE – THE INTUITIVE CREATIVE PRINCIPLE

In that the intuitive brain is the quiet, receptive part, it represents femininity in all of Creation. The creative impulse represents the masculine in is penetrative, fiery thrust, which, however, has to find its support for expression in the love of the fluid feminine.

Love is the feminine underlying principle of anything that is created. Love grants us the conscious enjoyment of our deep inner urges. Hence, womanhood represents the Law of Love in Creation, the transitional force through which the man's work is manifested. Her quiet weaving births all his creative ideation as she works in a helping way – strengthening, purifying, healing or even repelling.

For this reason the opening verse of the Creation Story according to Genesis begins: "And the spirit of God [the masculine executing force] moved upon the face of the waters [the feminine fluidity or womb]". Water symbolises procreation. Although as an element it appears calm and peaceful, when driven (by volition) water remains the most powerful, dominant and irresistible force, penetrating all species matter (mind) and fructifying it, cooling fire, and destroying anything that stands in its path. So is the power of woman.

The Story continues in verse 6 : "But there went up a mist from the earth, and watered the whole face of the ground". Symbolically, mist indicates an urge to conscious experiencing, condensation which produces precipitation – the preclusion to (pro)creation, thought-form. For this reason moisture is secreted by the procreative glands as the preparatory stage for the act of coition.

As the transitional or birthing force, woman therefore is the decisive factor, while the executing masculine energy is the fulfilment of all deeds in the field of objectivity. Only womanhood, as a privilege, has this higher spiritual nature – the transitional aspect behind the creating of form as a bridge within herself. Her more fluid intuitive perception makes her more accessible to the Creative Will of God, which manhood, the creative executive force, lacks.

This is woman's most precious secret within – intuitive perception. A force which is able to free the purity and sublimity of every thought, the inspiration to the greatest activity and noblest deed. This is providing, however, that she is the woman the Creator wanted her to be when he lavished these gifts upon her.

With her intuitive perceptions, woman is to support man. This sure is not a task for the species which is weaker. Whether it be mother, wife, friend, employee, employer, or admirer, she becomes his defender in shielding his back with her sharp physic senses, forever watchful and strengthening his efforts while he stands in the field of action.

As the stronger, more decisive factor, womanhood should strive to again take the lead if man is to ascend spiritually, this was and still remains her sacred duty. This role is something manhood needs to understand: that it rests with woman alone, through her spontaneity to go before him with purity in her soul and be his mediator of the creative radiations pulsating downward through the Universe.

This extended and more delicate ability of intuitive perception is woman's most precious gift of gifts, which no other creature can attain. Womanhood possesses within itself the strongest faculty towards the realisation of all that is good. Lying within this delicate sensitive vibration of intuitive perception is a fineness which holds the power to remodel everything in this world. Everything, from the crisis in world government, child poverty, to restoring the planet as a safe place to live psychically and physically. There is nothing that could resist this power if woman stands in her rightful place, for intuitive perception is connected to the Light and is therefore Life.

This help the man cannot do without if he wants to produce work of lasting value, for with his coarser nature he is not pervious enough to absorb these radiations himself. On his own, he cannot observe the intricate and delicate details of effective planning. Only when the man comes to this recognition will he be able to set goals with definite purpose, orderliness, precision, thoroughness and great organisational skill as well as the requisite deep intuitive knowing, to achieve lasting success.

Such activity, however, does not speak to the unnecessary exaggeration in the mad craving to accumulate riches or attain prominence in society. Such behavior not only upsets the necessary balance between rest and activity, but also prevents the necessary observance of the order of the home. Where one is inclined to such mania it can only lead to a life of high tension and stress-related illness and well as divorce. It only cultivates propensities of greed, avarice, acquisitiveness envy, *etc.*, never directed towards progress for humanity.

As long as the man's actions remain in the position of the intellect, where he is most comfortable, when confronted with delicate issues which require nurturing and sensitivity he will always be at a loss. This is why men suffer from feelings of inadequacy, because they are unfamiliar to tender emotions. Given his nature to take a stance, the warrior challenge is the most familiar position and he often moves into that mode of behavior.

Learning to work with the feminine principle will require great effort. However, if his highest endeavor is to strive to maintain balance in all Creation, before too long it will become second nature in the consciousness of his responsibility. He will no longer repress any tenderness when it comes to expressing emotion.

Working with the feminine, more spiritual principle demands clearing accumulated life experiences regarding his inappropriate use of power and preparing to step out of the false identity. It is a movement of total surrender and inner humility whereby he exposes "the ego" to a search at his every thought and volition; allowing him to shatter these destructive elements for a better understanding of himself.

His mind will gradually clear for the development and execution of his every act, whereas before, his thoughts were vague yielding unsatisfactory outcomes. He learns to intuitively weigh each step carefully and minutely against the objective, even if he has to revisit his plan of action at least ten times, so that his actions bring the desired conclusion.

His ability to observe this creative principle at work within himself or woman, becomes the doorway to his deeper levels of spiritual understanding as he utilises it to the fullest. As he develops this equanimity within himself, he finds little need for planning. That which comes to mind becomes "the done deed", for which Nature always provides the resources for fulfilment. For nought therefore it is said: *behind every successful man there stands a good woman* — whoever she is!

In this feminine support alone lies the man's self-respect. This is the secret between man and woman. That is what first makes every true man a man. From the fruit of his activity, man is able to respect himself when he can look up to womanly dignity. Only then does the urge arise within to protect that which gives him the respect for himself and upholds it – womanhood.

Then will the man see the activity of the woman in the household as just as important as his profession. He will no longer disregard the order of the household in an inconsiderate way, possibly through neglectful non-observance. He will see the woman's task in the home not merely as the one who ensures the health and vitality of his physical body in providing his meals and a comfortable place for recreation and rest, but so importantly... in providing *harmony among all souls who reside* in the home, which refreshes and offers a new incentive and strength for all his activities.

Hearth and Home

Where else is woman's most sacred place but "hearth and home"? This is the domain where she is respected in her most queenly aspect due to the nature of her activity.

Home is not to be understood as today's licensed institution where woman hires and sells herself simply to serve her husband, who does not seek in her a complimentary mate of equal worth, but who, apart from display, merely uses her as a cheap and willing housekeeper to make his home comfortable, and with whom he can also indulge his sexual appetite undisturbed and under the guise of respectability. Home speaks to her extended community and most importantly to the great household earth and its subsequent planes in this World of Matter, which offers her offspring subsistence to mature and come to ego-consciousness, not only to her matrimonial dwelling.

Woman's goal as determined from the beginning of time is to apply her exceptional creative ability to its uttermost heights in making this world a better place for all to live in. Not as wives and mothers basking in the achievements of their husbands, who offer them security as a dependent like a house built upon sinking sand. We witness this more today as woman sink deeper into poverty and low self-worth after divorce.

Every woman possesses what it takes to stand independently. She also dishonors herself through the delusion that she is supposed to consider motherhood as the principal purpose of her existence. Such false notion is the product of an ingrained social stigma upon her psyche where mistakenly she believes that she is expected to continue the primitive cycle of mother-animal, which is not her highest goal. By so doing she degrades herself in fulfilling the highest goal of the animal – childbearing.

This is a debasement of womanhood and a blow to humanity. For instead of pure sublime womanhood it is sacred motherhood and marriage. Motherhood is not a spiritual requirement, but that for which the animal instinct is needed. No matter how sacred motherhood becomes, the woman who submerges and looses herself in it cannot develop properly. Deceitfully she flatters her thoughts that motherhood is woman's highest task. But she is only confusing herself about her main vocation.

For thousands of years, this belief was so well encoded in us culturally that it forced the entire thinking of humanity in this direction. This endless cycle continues – producing offspring for the purpose of acquiring material things.

Married couples who are childless are described as barren, a curse placed upon them by society. Rather than adopt a child who needs a loving and caring family, they go to all lengths to conceive a child artificially.

Woman gets dragged into marriage too early, often before she has given thought to the purpose of her life and the skills she must develop to pursue her goals. Before long she finds herself frozen within her abilities at the time when the creative impetus of generative powers is most spontaneous.

Pursuing the path of wife and mother she squanders the entire strength her physical body, often holding down a full time job in the process. She becomes a mother without ever having been a real human being, before truly knowing herself. By the time her children are ready to leave home, there is no field left for her spirit to become active, she can no longer achieve something worthwhile.

The Battle of the Sexes

As we enter the new millennium, we hear more women declare that they are too astute for such oppression. They choose their mates of equal worth and feel no social pressure to bear children. However, their civil marriages remain nothing but sober business contracts in which the woman still binds herself. Although both parties regard it as a simple bargain ensuring each other's material security, if what follows is the surrendering of her body to her mate without further cogitation, is this not sexual bondage?

Astute as woman become, if marriage is not entered into for a spiritual harmony, it dishonors to both parties. It is impure and immoral – adulterous – even if sealed by civil law.

Social order cannot change the Natural Laws, which will never adapt themselves to human dispositions or to wrongly fostered ideas. The alarmingly high divorce rates and homosexual cohabitation point to social order gone wrong. Unless the state and social institutions adapt to the Laws of Nature, there will be no personal inner peace, much less peace and harmony between partners.

For womanhood to gain the respect and support of the man as well as her entire people, her base must again be "hearth and home". Many corporate women have already made the move back home. It is there her power lies. Not in public life where she did not belong in the first place, where she is forced to compete with man in the compelling, positive sphere of activity, that which Creation stipulated should remain purely masculine.

It is not that woman is not equal to man. She is – even stronger. But such fields of activity only harden her delicate intuitive perception through such struggle. Consequently, the highest ability and power which was bestowed upon her for her quiet weaving becomes exhausted. In the end, she coarsens or suppresses the delicate feminine altogether. In her ethereal body she sows this seed of her thoughts and actions, which geminates to bear fruit. What yields is a hybrid species or distorted soul – part female in body and part male energetically.

Today we find women driving heavy duty vehicles; taking front line positions on the battle front; (wo)manning construction sites; scaling utility poles; competing in high performance sports – all displaying developmental distortion in her brain. When the public of the City of Toronto around 1998 were asked to voice their opinions about police-public relation, they complained that female police officers were the most viscous towards civilians.

In a hardened psychic state, a woman can become more viscous than her male counterpart; for being the stronger species psychically, she now develops a coarseness which makes her more dominant and oppressive. Not only men complain of emasculation whether from mother, guardian or mate, but some women in homosexual relationships expose the brutal beatings from their mates. The finest thing when perverted, becomes the worst.

Any woman in this hardened condition repels anything that is genuine manhood. Her vigilante demeanor is but a facade trying to hide unquenchable feelings she bears in her soul of being misunderstood. In this disturbed equilibrium, she finds herself castrated in her own power, in her ability to change herself. This is the source of her constant unrest and often sadistic behavior.

This paralysis takes the form of a close embrace, silently suffocating her soul. Her real nature, which is naturally beautiful and exquisitely organised, because it is perverted, becomes proportionately ugly from her ill-disposition. Every now and then, in the midst of her oppressive delirium, her soul cries out to be freed, giving her insight as to how gravely internally oppressed and restrained she is in her movement to swing upward to her spiritual liberation through right action.

RECLAIMING FEMININITY

Feminine power emanates what is refined, more delicate and less dense. Bearing such quality, woman supplements human spirituality, holding it, as she stands to her appointed post in Creation. For this reason her body is not as strongly solidified as the man's, because this higher nature penetrates her more pervious ethereal body, which forms her physical body and keeps it loose.

This is not a deficiency nor a weakness sends women to exercise gyms toning every inch of her naturally loose body with high intensity equipment, but a necessity for the reception and mediation of radiations, the help of which man cannot do without. This makes woman stronger than man, psychically, not physically, for her power lies in her intuitive perception.

Coarseness is said to shrivel a woman's mammary glands. The noted 18th Century English physician warned, "The bosom is supplied with nerves of sensation from the cerebellum, and it is the most direct and intimate sympathy with the female generative organs. A woman of sensibility, who would preserve her chastity, must guard her bosom well." Only her loveliness and nurturing attributes can preserve her full bust.

The woman who represses her passive refined elements, loses them from lack of use. They gradually weaken and are drawn off by the same basic species. The passive feminine bridge needed to absorb higher radiations to be mediated to manhood and her descendants is subsequently broken. She therefore pushes man as well as her children to self-destruction, cut off form the Cosmic Light-Source (Life). She robs man of all that is sublime and prevents the flowering of noble manhood.

Thus it is said: *no nation or people can flourish and prosper, where the man is unable to look up to woman in her womanliness!*

The nation that subjects its women to these conditions, to strive towards the unsuitable state of manliness, will be sentenced to slow extinction. At first such wrong attitude brings difficult and premature child-birth. Through complicated child-birth, they issue children liable to all kinds of illness: anxiety and nervousness; deficient character; and torn intuitive perceptions (unstable minds). Finally, sterility is bound to set in within its women.

This is the main reason for youth delinquency and the low population growth among many of the so-called developed nations. Several generations will have to pass before the consequences of such an evil will be noticed, halted and corrected. Then will woman be able to restore her people from decline to a state of health and save itself from extinction; for with this changed inner psychic state, she will confer these elements on her offspring.

The woman who recognises such a distortion within her soul or who presently strives towards such a distortion can restore her true nature if she wants to. Her experience can help her to change; for she will notice that genuine men are never happy around her. They can never seem to understand her; because genuine manhood is repulsed by anything false, not to mention a woman striving to become man. A marriage of such sort is only an intellectual one, usually materialistically driven. They can never experience genuine love and harmony.

All such a woman has to do is suppress this distortion through a change in her mental attitude. She can purify her thoughts and perceptions by gaining an understanding of the Natural Laws and aspire to live them.

Since World War I, financial constraints have placed women in the sphere of work, occupying jobs which were predominantly male. The progression of this trend today poses the most devastating threat to the entire human. While many fear the devastating aftereffects of a World War III, the possibility of entire annihilation, they miss this brewing "battle of the sexes". Sole-support mothered households, the demand to make ends meet in a two-spouse household, the pressure of career and entrepreneurial ambition, leave woman little or no time to nurture her inherent delicate qualities.

Human existence will not cease with total annihilation by the atomic bomb. Though this can kill the body, it cannot kill the soul which reincarnates. When the male and female of earth fail to unite to again become that species which is perfect, through complimentary aggressive and passive activities, each split spirit-seed faces the possibility of dissolution. For within every immature seed lies the germ of death and decay.

Such a seed will eventually be lost along with the inherent possibility to become an independent fruit-bearing tree which, in turn, can help to continue the creative process of development – world without end – in higher ethereal planes beyond the third plane of human development. In other words, the spiritual personality it has acquired will be dissolved, so that it suffers spiritual death and disperses to primordial spirit-seed. It is not that extended opportunities could no longer be afforded the split germ-seed in its further development, but that the planet earth, being part of a Universe in the World of Matter which is now overripe, must disintegrate like every other planet that have completed its evolution to be formed anew.

Reaching the vortex of disintegration of all matter, under what condition can an unripe, that is, ethereally immature spirit-seed chain the lower three planes of existence fare? Non-belief in life after death cannot circumvent the law that no human spirit can ascend beyond its level of consciousness. Ones soul can only face unconsciousness due to the inability to withstand the higher pressure. The Law of Spiritual Gravity only pulls one of like species upwards to where it belongs.

The trends and impulses which today affect people and affairs is the transitional period for this renewal. Today there are only wars or rumors of war; auto immune diseases; upheavals becoming inevitable as the old passes. This is aftermath of the "battle of the sexes", the misuse of the masculine and feminine principles of Creation. The end will bring about the termination of the wrong principles, followed by the inner healing within the hearts of all humans.

Hence the great catastrophes today are but cleansing which becomes necessary for the earth to change. The last phase of the old and the beginning of the new show themselves in this transitional period in which current trends and impulses affect people and affairs.

The effects of this intense motion manifest in the extreme, not only in governmental affairs and other high places, but in marriages, family, social and business relations, as well as with one's self. The retroactive (karmic) effects of this final point of our actions and decisions now returns to us with superhuman speed and accuracy as we have never deemed possible here on earth. Every dark deed is exposed and collapses back upon its authors. At an alarming quick pace, we reap what we sow. Reprehensible wrongs, which long ago would stay hidden until long after one had died, are uncovered as those individuals with a "new" sense of decency and moral justice demand exposure and closure.

Only purity of intuitive perception can cultivate action to its crowning glory, heights undreamed of by any human mind. Its liberating effect engenders a keen sense of right and wrong, so no one need go astray. Only from this vantage point of perception can right and wrong be judged, not based on human rules of conduct but on the Natural Laws.

Developing the Ethereal Cloak

For the ethereal body to grow strong we must learn how to exercise intuitive perception. All it takes is to learn how to listen from that place of inner silence. This is called the "inner voice" – the spiritual part of us. The living human spirit expresses itself only and solely through intuitive perception. It is through the latter that the human spirit, the original spirit-seed evolved into a true "ego" due to the urge to taste of the "fruit of the tree of knowledge", to become active.

We can sense every pressure welling up within the ethereal cloak and learn to distinguish its assenting voice from that of our inner anxiety and fear and come to trust it. Our "gut" feeling, the first impression, is always right. This urging is equivalent to "knowing". Learning to "trust and obey" is the only way to happiness.

This demand, however, resting in the *Law of the Power of Every Simplification*, may offend the pride of many of us, due to the intellectual interpretation of such words rooted in our consciousness. But every movement up of intuitive perception is an event which radiates its effect into all the worlds and sinks upon milliard of smaller personalities, upon all that is objective. Until we "slay the dragon", that is, kill the lower "ego" of arrogance and conceit, we will remain unable to unfold our spiritual powers, to return to ourselves, to what we truly desire.

As we unremittingly attend to our l*ife's work and purpose*, we must also "give up ourselves", that is, surrender our vain would-be-knowledge, without contradiction and in a childlike manner, and devote ourselves to receiving spiritual powers intuitively. We must abort the "power trip" for that "transcendental trip" of intuitive perception. Then can we work with ethereal substance which, like the faculty of speech and action, is at our command.

In this manner alone do we gain the power to transform Nature, consequently quickening the spirit through experiencing, which brings understanding. Not the pitiable state in which many of us engage intuitive perception as absorbing experiences outside of us whether through observation or learning, and transform them for further development and maturity of the spirit. Both functions of intuitive activity should be operational.

This process reveals our true nature. Good and evil are reinforced and animated by our spiritual power, which is a "neutral power". This power, however, does not reside in the being, but works only through one's intuitive perception. In this, each of us determines the nature of volition. Spiritual power brings good or evil, it is sheer power which vitalises whatever is willed.

Each of us is merely a guardian of this creative power, which works in accord with our volition. We must therefore act as good custodians at the door of our soul, ready to be held accountable for all activities therein, every moment of the day.

Instead of unquenchable desire for sensual fulfilment, we now learn to perceive the workings of animistic and ethereal substance within our being and this will create the right emptiness for the vastness of Nature to fill. This does not mean we must constantly observe each and every happening intellectually, that would be to stand beside our intuitive perception. It is like living with two personalities. Although we bear within us the capacity to perceive and understand, at times, we become arrogant and conceited. The latter develops from the quest for self-esteem, it kindles and nourishes such passions and hinders every genuine experience, ultimately severing the faculty of intuition. We only dissipate valuable generative power in this intellectual game.

While the faculty of observation remains the only door through which knowledge enters the mind, intuitive perception is the key to open our capacity for observation, which helps us adapt to the mighty Laws of Nature operating within the powerful emissions of our elemental faculties. Only when we study and adapt ourselves to the special nature of these powers within ourselves will we begin to feel at home with Mother Nature, and not like foreign microbes, destroying every harmony of Her great household. Such destructiveness must be expelled if health is to be restored to this planet.

Equally important, we will learn to convert our present sexual and marital sufferings into enjoyment. By expounding and applying Nature's sexual ordinances to our lives, as well as diet and lifestyle among other things, we align head and heart; body and soul; the material and the spiritual. Before long we will be able to perceive the delicate reflections of our ethereal body, and observe all that is to be revealed to us in our surroundings for our self-perfection.

As we observe and study – without judgement – our surroundings, people and their behavior, we see reflections of our own unique nature and life mysteries that reveal themselves to us. Then will the joy gained form the fulfilment of our desires and actions lift us to that conscious existence where we experience pure bliss.

As explained, the spirit is human's innermost core which controls the animation of our intuitive perceptions and thoughts. For the spirit's radiation to come into contact with its outside surroundings, it needs a bridge, and this radiation bridge is the astral body – our emotions.

The astral bridge connects the radiation of the spirit to its surroundings by its invisible navel cord, which in its natural state is said to be of a silvery sheen and of a finer substance than the navel cord at birth. This allows the spirit's radiation to project beyond the physical body in what is called the aura. When this "silver cord" is broken, death occurs, and the physical body and spirit separates. The so-called ghost or shadow remains visible to some, which is the astral cloak.

The nerve centre of the solar-plexus connects with the frontal brain via the intuitive back-brain through special nerve paths along the spinal cord. Hence the astral bridge is the final link between spirit and matter (brain). One part of this bridge leads away from the conscious brain with our formed expression of thoughts and actions back to the spirit; the other part leads to the brain from the spirit, which stimulates it with inspirations and inventions – whatever it takes to bring about the fulfilment of desires.

Leading away from the brain, the spiritual act of unification and condensation produces new thought-forms. Through union, our thoughts and actions form bridges that receive influx of higher thoughts called inspiration.

Thought-power

Union presses the elements of thoughts and actions into service to mature in their perfection. The fructified thought will be attracted to, and itself attract, those of similar nature, and contact a power-centre identical to the nature of the thought. In the process it receives increased power through the reciprocal action. Union moulds, refines and forms in the process called fusion; the process wherein forms undergo transformation through the pressure of varied elements, in this case, the attraction of other thought-forms to produce a perfectly new thought-form which is then directed back as inspirations to the brain via the astral body.

Now effective through reciprocal action, the original thought brings calmness, strength, recovery, plans and solutions suddenly arising in the brain. As long as it is a powerful, uplifting thought, something good will always come of it, be it only a stabilising of mind, which leads to some way out of a difficulty. It is also possible that the original thought will find an ethereal path to people who, being stimulated through this, will bring about a fulfilment.

There is, however, one impediment to the fulfilment of thought-volition which causes us to encounter failure and non-fulfilment. Though sometimes we feel we are clear as to what we are about, even with the best and greatest desire, within us there usually remains reservation - a fear which causes hesitation to access the fullness and prosperity embedded in each volition. This reservation is about the lower self, the "ego" with its lack of confidence and trust, which rises unconsciously and causes our thinking to be rigid. It resists the fluidity, the spontaneity, of the intuitive creative process. Combined with our subconscious belief systems, we suppress the power of thought with a clinging tenacity.

The "ego" keeps itself hidden, sending out harmful feelings of inadequacy and unworthiness, cynicism, distrust, doubt, fear, guilt, superstition, irresolution, timidity, procrastination, fault-finding, contrariety, and many other forms of negativity when we least expect them. It obtrudes itself in many things, especially when decisions must be made on the spot, even hindering the fulfilment of desire completely. Although this obtrusion occurs temporarily - when the volition towards fulfilment is strong, it nevertheless weakens the effect of the will to fulfil, and delays many a success, hindering it or making it quite impossible.

Incoming impressions can also be evil thoughts sent to us and can soil us as if mud and dirt were thrown at us, if our thoughts and perceptions are likewise impure or we are not so morally strong. Over time, we may become confused under this barrage. This happens because impure thought-forms cling to our aura and attract other people's thoughts of like nature, strengthening them. They may linger until that very moment when the nature of our own thoughts become of like manner, then they saturate our bombarded soul like an injection of poison.

One with a disturbed or diseased brain may even be compelled to commit the most gruesome crime such as murder which, under normal circumstances, the perpetrator would not possess the spiritual vigour to develop one's own thoughts strongly enough to become a powerful act. This has led so many to flock to psychotherapists; also to disciples of occult science for psychic help, visits born of fear that another has cast a spell over them, or that they themselves seek to cast a spell.

In that each thought-form bears power and life within, which continues to develop and work in the desired direction, how an evil thought will affect the other person to whom it is sent depends on the psychic condition of the one concerned. It may bring much or little harm, perhaps even different from what was intended, or none whatsoever. One's inner psychic condition is the governing factor, thus no one is exposed to such power unprotected.

Impressions entering the solar plexus radiate upon the heart, sometimes strongly enough to be felt and stamped with personal ownership, thus leaves "lasting impression". We say we learn from an experience. In this also lies the meaning of the expression: "to take to heart." The same goes for every act of willing. It awakens the intuitive perception as powerful waves of emotion within the solar plexus with its ganglion of the sympathetic nerve branches lying beneath the diaphragm.

This is why we cannot think straight when there is solar plexus crisis whether it be the experience of some deep emotion which gives "butterflies" or distress of the digestive system. All attention is then focused on that deep (intuitive) "gut feeling", which proves therefore, that the intuitive brain is the leading brain and that the solar plexus is where we experience things. The gut is a mind of its own upon which the intellectual brain remains dependent.

The intellectual brain can only do so much before it tires and must rest if it is to remain functional. The intuitive brain, however, receives impressions or influences from the inside as well as from the outside world; receives dreams; regulates the digestive process with its network of nerve cells surrounding our digestive system after the frontal brain finishes its active role and rests.

Action is the resultant reception from the intuitive brain which the intellect transmits. And when the brain has finished its task, for example eating, the intuitive brain which never rests, continues the digestive process unconsciously.

THE SMALL (INTUITIVE) BRAIN AS AFFECTING MENTALITY

The astral body (emotions) controls, directs and moves the physical body through the intuitive brain (cerebellum). It is it's spiritual prototype from which the human body is formed. This is why if the spirit and the body do not swing in harmony in the field of action, the latter will not be maintained and strengthened through its work, but become worn and exhausted through growing tension, because it does not receive the spiritual strength it needs through the mediation of the animistic faculties. The intensification or weakening of our emotions determines body "weight", astrally. Expression of our emotions in the fulfilment of activity makes us feel light; a weakening from non-expression makes us feel heavy.

Obesity and anorexia are more the result emotional disturbances than organic factors, in that whatever happens to the astral body is also suffered by the physical body. The sufferings of the physical body, however, touch the astral body much less, even though they are connected.

Spiritual stagnation hampers the full development of the physical body. In the end, the body consumes itself. It can no longer regenerate because its source – the spiritual – is lacking.

Neuroscience confirms that the growing cause of tension in the body stems from the emotional level. And regeneration can only begin there.

Practicing self-control manipulates our neuromuscular mechanism which is dual in nature, *i.e.*, capable of reacting in two ways - voluntary and involuntary. Voluntary reactions contribute to movements which catch the eyes more readily than involuntary movements, say of heat or cold, attraction or repulsion. These natural movements determine the body's posture, and gives it its muscle tone.

How the frontal brain develops naturally influences the forming of the physical body. Like distorted sexuality, those individuals who at birth bear within the soul the propensity to develop themselves in a purely intellectual way, in this case they possess frontal part of the brain that is disproportionately enlarged. This has led scientists to refer to the back brain as the "small brain". The science of phrenology was established on the grounds that the development of the human form is reflective of the formation of the brain, which affects mentality. The following position on the size of the brain was taken by O.S. Fowler:

> Size, other things being equal, indicates the power of function, that this proportion expresses a general law, is evinced by the general fact that the larger the pieces of wood, iron, *etc.*, are, the stronger they are; the larger horses, persons, *etc.*, are stronger, can lift, draw, and endure more than smaller, and thus of everything else. Though sometimes smaller men, horses, *etc.*, are stronger, can lift, draw, and endure more than others that are larger, because they are different in organic quality, health *etc.*, yet where the quality is the same, whichever is the largest is proportionally the most powerful.
>
> And this undisputed law of things is equally true of the brain, and that mental power put forth from it. All really great men [and women] have great heads – merely smart ones, or those great only in certain faculties or specialties of character, not always.... The heads of Washington,

> Adams, and a thousand celebrities, were also very large. Bright, apt, smart, literary, knowing, even eloquent men and women *etc.*, often have only average, even moderate-sized heads, because endowed with the very highest organic quality, yet such are more admired than commanding; more brilliant than powerful; more acute than profound. Though they may show off well in an ordinary sphere, yet they are not the men and women for great occasions; nor have they the giant force of intellect which molds and sways nations and ages. The phrenological law is, that size, other things being equal, is a measure of power; yet these other conditions, such as activity, power, motive, health, physiological habits, *etc.*, increase or diminish the mentality even more than size. Quality is more important than quantity, but true greatness requires both cerebral quantity and quality.
>
> Still, those again who large heads, are sometimes dull, almost foolish, because their organic quality is low. As far, then, as concerns Phrenology itself, this doctrine of size appertains to the different organs in the same head, rather than to different heads. Still this doctrine, that size in the measure of power, is no more a special of Phrenology than of every other department of nature. And those who object to this science on this ground are objecting to a known law of things. If size were the only condition of power, their cavils might be worthy of notice; as it is, they are not.[9]

The doctrine of phrenology shows in every respect the continuous and uninterrupted working upward of the Creative Will in Nature; a proof of the perfection of Creation. A development proceeding downward produces the opposite effect and grotesque deformities in both brain and body.

Importantly, the doctrine also declares, head shape does not necessarily go hand in hand with the development of spiritual self-consciousness in the body. This is the aspect of the philosophy which is in line with the principle of body alignment which, does not give credence to the doctrine of superiority of any group whether by race or class by the size and shape of the head. None is below and above another, every human being is equally valuable and therefore an indispensable member of the human race, and just as important is one's contribution to society in the fulfilment of their *life's work and purpose*. The different races have their material and spiritual values which are complimentary, and belong absolutely to the growth and prosperity of that particular people. As Gellert stated, "You do not have what others have, and others lack your gifts; from this deficiency springs good fellowship" (Fables, "The Blind Man and the Lame Man").

The turmoil of experiencing – the pain, disappointments, grief – which is a necessity, is the sole help for us to see our mistakes and imperfections to correct them, and is the only way to gain self-consciousness. It is our imperfection we are here to transmutate into perfection, in order to fit into divine ordinances of things – if we are to experience any form of love, joy, peace and happiness, as we learn and understand the Natural Laws.

As long as one sets out on the path to self-improvement, no matter if one is a criminal or of low intelligence, in cultivating those faculties that are weak with the right mental stimulation and correct choice of nutrients, it is the ethereal body not the body form that is subject to this new development. The latter is subject only to limited changes. Thus phrenological indications may outwardly appear normal or abnormal, well developed or underdeveloped; whereas at the level of the soul, the converse is true. However, the following observations are worth some attention.

Body Language

According to Fowler:

> A head projecting far back behind the ears, and hanging over and downward in the occipital region, indicates very strong domestic and social affections, a love of home, its relations and endearments, and a corresponding capacity of being happy in the family, and having a happy family. The social affections are located in the back part of the

head; and accordingly, woman being more loving than man, when not under the influence of the other faculties, usually inclines her head backward, and when she kisses children, and those she loves, always turns the head directly backward, and rolls it from side to side, on the back of the neck.

Wide and round heads, on the contrary, indicate strong animal and selfish propensities, while thin, narrow heads indicate a corresponding want of selfishness and animality. A head projecting far up at the crown indicates an aspiring, self-elevating disposition, pride of character, and a desire to be and to be something great; while a flattened crown indicates a want of ambition, energy and aspiration. A head high, long, and wide upon the top, but narrow between the ears, indicates Casuality (planning, thinking, reason, sense), moral virtue, much practical goodness, and a corresponding deficiency of these humane and religious susceptibilities. A head wide at the upper part of the temples indicates a corresponding desire for perfection, together with a love of the beautiful and refined, while narrowness in this region evinces a want of taste, with much coarseness of feeling.

Fullness over the eyes indicates excellent practical judgement of matters and things appertaining to property, science, and nature in general; while narrow, straight eyebrows indicate poor judgement of matter, things, their qualities, relations, and uses. Fullness from the root of the nose upward indicates great practical talent, love of knowledge, desire to see, and ability to say and do the right thing at the right time, and in the best way, together with sprightliness of mind; while a hollow in the middle of the forehead shows off to advantage. A bold, high forehead indicates strong reasoning capabilities, while retiring forehead indicates less soundness, but more availability of talent. And thus of the cerebral developments.

Phrenology teaches that every faculty, when active, moves head and organ in the direction of the acting organ. Thus intellect, in the fore part of the body, moves it directly forward, and produces a forward, hanging head. Hence, intellectual men never carry their heads backward and upward, but always forward; and logical speakers move their heads in a straight line, usually forward toward the audience; while vain speakers hold their heads backward. Hence it is a poor sign to stand so straight as to lean backward, for it shows that the brain is in the wrong place – more in the animal than intellectual region. Perceptive intellect, when active, throws out the chin and lower portion of the face; while reflective intellect causes the upper portion of the forehead to hang forward, and draws in the chin, as in Franklin, Webster, and other great thinkers. A coxcomb once asking a philosopher, What makes you hang your head down so? Why don't you hold it up as I do? was answered: "Look at that field of wheat! The heads that are well filled bend downward, but those that stand up straight are empty." Benevolence throws the head and body slightly forward, leaning toward the object which excites its sympathy; while Veneration causes allow bow, which, the world over, is taken as respect; yet, when Veneration is exercised toward the Deity, a sin devout prayer, it throws the head upward; and, as we use intellect at the same time, the head is generally directed forward.

He who meets you with a long, low bow thinks more of you than of himself; but he who greets you with a short, quick bow – who makes half a bow forward, but a bow and a half backward – thinks one of you, and one and a half of himself. Ideality throws the head slightly forward and to one side such as one gifted in taste and imagination as any other writer. Very firm men stand straight up and down, inclining not a hair's breath forward or backward, or to the right or left; hence the expression "He is an up-and-down man." And this organ is located exactly on a line with the body. Self-esteem, located in the back and upper portion of the head, throws the head and body upward and backward. Large feeling, pompous persons walk in a very dignified, majestic manner, throwing their heads backward, but to one side. The difference between the natural language of these two organs is so slight that only [the keenest observer] can perfectly distinguish them.

The natural language of Money-loving, carries the head forward and to one side, as if in ardent pursuit of something, and ready to grasp it with outstretched arms; while Alimentiveness (appetite, relish, greediness) situated lower, hugs itself down to the dainty dish with the greediness of an epicure, better seen than described. The shake of the head is the natural Language of Combativeness, and means "No I resist you." Those who are combating earnestly shake the head more or less violently, according to power of the combative feeling, but always shake it slightly inclining backward; while Destructiveness, inclining forward, causes a shaking of the head slightly forward, and turning to one side. When a person who threatens you shakes his head violently, and holds it partially backward, and to one side, never fear – he is only barking; but whoever inclines his head to one side, and shakes it violently, will bite, whether possessed of two legs or four. Thus it is with each of the various postures assumed by individuals express the relative activity, present or permanent, or their respective faculties...[10]

Posture and Its definition

Posture may be defined as an attitude assumed by the body either (i) with support, during muscular activity or (ii) the co-ordination of several muscles to (a) to maintain stability or (b) form an essential basis for any movement, this basis adapted constantly to the type of movement, super-imposed on it.

With this definition clear, we only have to observe the posture of those whose body does not swing with spirit, where the thought-power governs bodily actions and not the power of intuitive perceptions. The posture of a gymnast is a classic example. When she is not on "stage", if we observe how she sits, stands, and walks, we see how deplorable her posture often becomes.

This points to the fact that her strength and suppleness with a grace of movement is of the physical body alone; and that she only developed physical strength needed to support her posture when performing, which calls for enormous nervous tension. Only a few show the stability of continual co-ordination of all muscles as generated by the astral body in their daily activities.

Observe other athletes also. Their walk is very often anything but beautiful, their carriage seldom graceful. You will see that they are far from controlling their bodies. The reflexive behavior of posture is not fine and automatic neuromuscular activity. Their heavy ponderous steps show anything but delicate intuitive-power.

A body which is maintained and permeated by spiritual power has fluid movements and strides, along with a light, springy step regardless of its weight. It is like a bow and arrow. If the bow is high-strung, the arrow overshoots its mark.

It is of this "high strung" experience most athletes suffer, a condition that heightens their reflex activity, wasting generative power in maintaining a contraction of muscles. Fatigue occurs so easily and there is no real experience of rest, even when they try to relax or sleep. Many athletes, even at the peak of their careers, find it hard to slow down, much less quit, so as to try to find harmony with the variance they have set up within their bodies.

This is not to underestimate the invaluable effect of yogic style exercises, brisk walking or chiropractic manipulations, The benefits are clear especially in cases of neurosis with accompanying psycho-physical tensions.

Invaluable are these approaches in cases where there is constant fatigue from growing bodily tension. They help attain and maintain homeostasis in the mental as well as the physical. To gain lasting effects, those who are so affected must be willing to work on themselves emotionally. With mere physical exercises and manipulations, clinical observations reveal that even with the so-called normal, there are subconscious patterns which require a considerable amount of effort to overcome inertia to change. "They are slow to react completely, reach maximum effectiveness gradually, and also subside slowly".

EMOTIONS AND THE DEVELOPMENT OF POSTURE

The variance between body and spirit can only be harmonised by the intuitive back-brain, the central organ of all orderly movements of the traverse muscular system for maintaining the tension of muscles and the balance of the body. The intuitive brain, in receiving information from all parts of the body, makes instant decisions, thereby controls and improves all movements.

Although the frontal brain regulates the nerve-stimuli to the physical organ for the completion of a movement, the intuitive back-brain fine tunes the movement. It corrects the actual posture of the body, with regard to the position of the limbs, the speed of movement, and the influences of the force of gravity.

"Mind over matter" (body) becomes evident in the grace and beauty of one's movements, a display of a harmonious working of the intuitive and the intellectual brains. Whenever pure emotions completely permeate and control the physical body through the intuitive brain, beauty is bound to show in our movements, it cannot do otherwise. The physical senses also become permeated with beauty, so that we ennoble everything we do.

Postural beauty and grace are the expressions of a pure human spirit in all its activities; a combined harmonious co-operation between the front and back brains. Physical exercises, gymnastics and other extravagances have little influence on the body, except for their residual effect. Without the integrated cultivation of pure emotions, that is, desires void of self-aggrandisement, we take ponderous steps, at a high metabolic cost. Those with heavy steps prove lack of proper mastery of their bodies through their spirit.

An efficient posture is defined as one that fulfils in the most economic way the purpose of the specific activity for which it serves as

a background, *i.e.*, which involves no unnecessary muscular effort for its maintenance and adjustment. An efficient posture develops naturally provided the inherent mechanisms are healthy and intact, with adequate tone in the muscles involved.
To control the body energetically all day, requires radiant strength. But this can only be supplied from *inner spiritual power*, from which the body can derive up to ten times more benefit than that which comes from these outside stimuli of gymnastics and other postural manipulations.

Spiritual control distinguishes humans from animals, which are subject to different laws. The animal fulfils these laws, its body and soul harmonise, and its movement always shows a beauty adapted to its body. In contrast to humans, it has a light step despite its physical weight, which is often enormous.

A trip to the zoo, or better yet, any wild life sanctuary, brings this contrast home. Unless limited by some ailment, the movement of animals are absolutely "natural", while those of *humans* lack the harmony between body and soul. Humans merely hobble, or rather, stomp along, either thoughtlessly or in deep thought, or hasten nervously, distraught and absentminded. There is no beauty at all, which one would envision in the meaning of the words, "to stride" and "to walk".

Language and The Emotions

Language was developed out of the need to express the deep emotions of the soul. Hence in the astral plane lies our oneness with all other human beings, where we share a common background of interpretation. On the astral level we live together in language, no matter the race, colour, creed or tongue. We all cry, laugh, feel hungry, loved or unloved.

This emotional homogeneity gives us all the capability to understand, communicate and work with each other. Although words develop from this plane, one does not have always to speak to send a message. The message can be picked up in our moods and emotions. Whether we are verbal or not, our emotions are felt by others, through our body language.

Emotions of joy, happiness and confidence stimulate and keep an alert posture, in which positions of extension predominate. Unhappiness, mental conflicts, and feelings of inadequacies and inferiority give rise to the condition of flexion with the head bent down, curling forward, and chest sunken inward. Anger causes the body to stretch to its full height, but with a disturbance in the muscle tone it gives rise to tremors. Fear increases this disturbance to tottering. Extreme terror makes one's body flop, with no tone in the muscles at all.

Words In Motion

At times, especially in today's business dealings, we try to hide our true emotions behind our words. In the end this will not only betray but destroy us, if only our public image.

Our deceptive nature sets up a dichotomy in our conscious or unconscious reactions, for the astral body sends this message to every cell of the body. Deception, or any other vices can never hide behind words, no matter how hard we try; for in the Law of Reciprocal Action (karma) they continuously design the public identity we wish to build for our weakness. It paints the false picture by which we continue to deceive and reassure ourselves about our own shortcomings, hence our pseudo-personalities.

Although with free will we are able to form our words, like everything else our words are motives and send out active rays and are active. With words we build our kingdoms, *i.e.*, conditions in life which we attract to ourselves.

Words are astral-forms which give rise to incisive effects upon those around us. Our words determine if we are looked upon as sincere or insincere. With every urge to say something our intuitive perception becomes more strengthened and automatically produces an astral form which embodies the nature of our true intention. As our intuitive perception rises higher and finally reaches the brain, it excites thoughts of similar nature, which we form into "stories" to influence others.

Irrespective of our real intention behind our imaginative stories, words themselves (with their own interpreted forms) have generative power; their own meaning, separate from the intention of the speaker. It is the generative power of the word itself that acts upon the listener. If the currents set in motion by words of the speaker bring about contrary elements on this homogenous astral level of any listener, there can be no support for what is being said, and, to the keen observer, the speaker reveals his insincerity.

In the astral body around the physical body of the speaker, invisible but felt, the ethereal cloak births a dark grotesque form which corresponds with the manner of such deceptive thoughts and actions. The form resembles the speaker, his true ugly nature, for it is the child of our volition that issued from him. This is why we find that such individuals are often repulsed by others of lighter and purer minds though they may not be able to put a finger on the reason for distrust; whereas they find affinity with those of the same dark or indolent minds. Hence it is said "you are the crowd you keep".

For those whose thoughts and emotions are of a purer and finer nature as their delicate ethereal cloak, their aura bears light around them and attracts only those individuals of like mind. The light of the soul, the aura, depends upon the ethereal cloak for the absorption of rays of Light penetrating down through the Universe.

The more ethereal our thoughts and perceptions, *i.e.*, of less materialistic and sensual emotions, the purer and more uplifting will be our surroundings. Our presence will always bring light. As it is said: we "light up" the place. We do not have to make our presence known where ever we go, we are felt the minute we walk into a room. There is an instant attraction. Our altered DNA also emanates in an enhanced physical appearance.

The reason for this, as already said, is that the radiation of the species of matter most strongly represented is that which naturally predominates in our actions. And that which predominates will in turn exert the greatest influence upon the inside as well as upon the outside.

So when the ethereal body predominates, our colour-radiations attract and absorb those same radiations. We emanate colours vibrating emotions of peace, joy, happiness and bliss in our immediate environment, based on the nature of our thoughts, perceptions and works. It all lies in the power of attraction. Hence the colour of one's clothing and personal surroundings indicate the nature of his soul, for colour determines the species the same as the species determines the colour.

Emanating such qualities from the soul implies that one is also more knowledgeable, more creative and wiser than others with a more dense brain due to their heavier, more materialistic concerns of darker radiations. For due to easier receptivity of one's ethereal cloak, the lighter soul is able to experience in the time of a day what it takes others a year, or even years, to achieve.

This is so evident in language. When the intention of our soul does not simultaneously vibrate with words, it either glitters like sham gold, too good to be true for the not-so-gullible; or like heavy, depressing grey clouds if they are filled with incomprehensibilities and amplifications.

For this reason we are only to speak the truth, no matter the cost, if we must. But making sure, however, that our speech creates no disharmony in the atmosphere. We must heed our words, *i.e.*, speak what we truly experience inside. The marketing and promotional pitches bombarding us subliminally in order to sell products and services, are but carefully crafted stories designed to deceive. They will not succeed with the intuitively astute.

Words were not meant to be uttered for the sake of talking, but for the expression of that which is necessary for the soul. Words are meant to direct the heart's desires, mapping a path for the way the intuitive perception wants to go. At the same time, forming in part a signpost indicating the direction of the rays of intuitive perception, while keeping certain types of intuitive perception together so as to envisage more clearly through words.

Jesus admonished: *let your communication be yea or nay; for what is more than these cometh evil.* Every spoken word should reflect the splendor of the Creative Word in the beginning: Let there be Light! Human words are but tiny reflections, though faint, of the Light of God.

We will only reap evil consequences of hardships, failures and diseases if we are insincere with our words; for corresponding to the evil returning karma is the stressful impingement of the grosser immune system, which is connected to the aura to protect the physical body. The nature of our thoughts, intuitive perception, words, and actions, be they good or evil, determine the strength or weakness of the protective mechanism of the immune system.

Like the network of nerves surrounding the digestive system, which according to Dr. Michael Gershon,[II] "resembles basketball netting, with the hoop being our digestive tract"[II], so the returning evil karma is woven into the astral body in what is called "threads of fate" as emotional blocks which lead to digestive disturbance and related diseases, or at least a tendency toward this.

THE INTELLECT – "THE SERPENT"

The intellect is the highest power in the World of Matter; the steering element, that is, that which serves purely to make movement possible in fulfilling our *life's work and purpose*. But the intellect can also become the serpent, challenging the spirit's decision not to eat "the apple", of the tree of good and evil, the tree of the quest for purely intellectual knowledge and the things of this world in its pursuit of knowledge if we expect to come to "ego-consciousness". If we yield to its persuasions, in the end we only find ourselves thrust pitilessly on the road to destruction, cut off from real life, plagued with all kinds of mundane and health problems.

Such is the nature of the intellect, because it is earthbound. Issued from the brain which is subject to matter, it cannot ascend to what is spiritual. Lacking such ability it can never bring understanding, an intuitive seeing or hearing, much less investigate or classify spiritual things for earthly conceptions. Only in the intuitive-spiritual perception can this happen.

To elevate the intellect to the position reserved for the spirit brings in its wake the natural consequence that, over time, such cultivation and activity causes the brain to strengthen one-sidedly. And this wrong attitude mankind has engaged itself in for thousands of years.

The consequence now shows itself in a distortion whereby that part which must do all the work – the cerebrum – grows bigger than the other part, the small cerebrum brain, which subsequently becomes stunted. According to phrenology, the increase of one portion of the brain more than another elevates that portion of the skull above it; for the shape of the brain determines the shape of the skull, and with a few exceptions, corresponds to it. Therefore, a large skull is not necessarily a recommendation, but may indicate an excessive strain to which the frontal brain *alone* has been subjected, which has fostered human development far beyond everything else. In the natural course of things, one fault brought the other in its train, which ultimately brought about the what is called the "fall of man", in the allegory of the Tower of Babel.

Hence the debate as to the amount of blood that is sent to the brain in proportion to the other parts of the human system. All agree that the brain consumes more blood relative to any other part. Some say it uses five times, some say eight, others, up to twenty times more than other parts based on demand. According to Fowler, "the difference between them can only be attributed to the difference in the talents of those experimented upon, intellectual subjects having the most ... The distinctiveness and protrusion of the veins in the blood of great men, and also the immediate filling up of these veins when one laughs or becomes excited, have the same cause."

So today our spirit lies in its physical body as if in a sack tied at the top by the intellect. Consequently, we have failed to mature in keeping rhythm with the entire Worlds of Matter and have allowed our ethereal bodies to decay. Disease has ensued in the physical body and we are unable to gain control over our own personal lives and affairs. All because we have voluntarily abandoned the prescribed course for our development. We concentrated all our energy upon training the intellect in a one-sided manner, carving our instrument – the brain – into our idol.

The frontal brain, having now become the producer, is forced to overexert itself to meet the needs of the other bodily instruments. Yet for harmonious activity, like everything in the body, both parts of the human brain should develop absolutely *equally*. The spirit taking the lead; while the intellect executes the effects in the field of relativity. Since this is not the case, the activity of the body, and even the body itself, is not be what it should be. For what has taken place affects everything.

Childhood Development

The result of over-cultivation of the intellectual brain is what is called, the "hereditary sin". That is, in time, the over-cultivation of our now deformed frontal brain, called the large brain, was inherited by each child.

Thank goodness this does not mean humanity has inherited the sin itself, but only the danger. From birth, those so dispositioned inherit the tendency to excessively and artificially cultivate the otherwise called "great brain" which makes them vulnerable, too easily entangling themselves in evil doings.

We witness this in children today who are born with an increasingly developed and stronger frontal brain – called the "whiz kids". Culminated from the wrong schooling, at an early age their intellect begins its one-sidedly development. From a tender age already the physical cloak around the spirit is kept closely tied, so that it simply cannot come to development or gain authority.

Intellectually driven men and women design curricula for childhood education, which is but one-sided and lacking in spiritual balance. It encourages mental prodigies instead of plenty of physical training. Children are not allowed to develop at their own pace, learn by doing instead of remembering. Subsequently, they do not develop independence, self-reliance nor self-government; virtues which induce the spirit to act responsibly and account for their conduct. Children should have short school days where they do a great deal of play and fresh air. Instead of a working of the animistic forces of Nature to explore the natural development of all life in our natural surroundings and appreciate such wonders, subjects of study entail only rigid dogma forced upon the spirit at this vulnerable age to produce super kids.

Such learning cannot kindle the spirit towards its own free conviction about what is really important in life, because the natural foundation is lacking. It is vain, bears no vitality and has no connection to the spiritual-creative aspect of mind but only to that of the conceit of intellectual advancement. Even in such institutions where childhood education is not so one-sided, where teachers employ empirical knowledge with respect to character analysis to understand each pupil instead of forcing and drilling the child, because of the genetic disposition of a large frontal brain, the spirit remains too feeble to keep pace with the intellect, which has now grown so strong.

By the onset of adolescence, the animistic bridge from the spirit to our natural environment is hindered, the path fallen or crumbling. Hence we find youth today cut off from all loving spiritual activity which animates and inspires the intellect. A duality results within their innermost self and many teenagers seek suicide as the way out. The child, however, who through this wrong development continues on this path into adolescence, is only partly to be blamed. All those involved in his or her education and training must bear part of the fault, because they helped this one-sided lush growth. In the Law of Reciprocal Action, from that first moment of training onwards they are connected to the child until it is freed from this mistake and its consequences, until the child so educated has had the opportunity to consider and retrace its steps. Such opportunities never fail to come, no matter how rude the awakening.

Unfortunately, in the majority of cases, the intellectual gulf between the two parts of the human brain has grown so wide and the functions so disproportionate, an improvement can no longer be achieved without painful experiences in life.

The Oppressive Male

A spiritual inadequacy creates within the male the desire for dominance and the repression of any tenderness when it comes to feelings. Hence the male's ever insensitivity towards the female, because his feeling is not guided by the delicate intuitive perception of his spirit.

The impressions predominantly meant for his spirit can only be absorbed by his intellect, and bounded without being able to penetrate to the spirit. His spirit receives nothing and the intellect everything.

Thus the condition is finally reached when the spirit is no longer capable of absorbing anything at all. Robbed of the ability to receive impulses from the radiations of the Universe, to the *spirit-part* comes to a standstill, hence an inclination to spiritual inactivity. He can only experience blockage to his creative expression, giving rise to errors and poor judgement.

By the time the youth begins to perform tasks he should and develop properly as a human being, his spirit is already stunted and smothered by the weight of this dross. There only remains an unquenchable yearning to give some inkling of the presence of his immured and suppressed spirit. Finally even this longing is lost in the mad whirl of haste and greed which is first meant as a bridge over this spiritual vacuum, and which later becomes a habit and a need.

The best the intellectually driven male can produce are "weak-hearted" or "heart-less" conceptions – insensitivity towards the plight of human sufferings. He finds himself totally incapable of engaging in deep sensitive issues, utterly remote from his capacity to understand.

Unconditionally, he is left with no choice but to submit himself to his own intellectual thinking. Incapable of grasping anything that is spiritual, he cannot help but entangle himself in all sorts of evil which is inevitable when the intellect dominates. In this mode he carries a corresponding deformed dense brain which narrows the range of his perceptive capacity to the purely material things of life. He only lives a minute part of his real existence, unable to think outside of structured reality.

Sad but true, the majority of these men and woman-man represent power, from government to the religious institutions. Their imagination aids them to become these fictional characters, of boastful conceit, commercialism, morbid imagination and hypocrisy, in the craving for power and earthly admiration created out of the sultry swamp of their base narrow-mindedness.

Some prize themselves as proud materialists, which of course, is no applause, but evidence of their deformed brain. It only shows a limitation which in their arrogant lust for power, their self-centeredness, distrust and the never-ending disputes among themselves. They become not only a danger to themselves, but to the rest of society. They act and pass legislation without heart. Their feeling follows a narrow funnel through the retrospective effect of their calculating thinking.

And from troubled brains what do we get? The troubled economies of the world today. Social and economical problems which will never be solved in the distortions of today's patriarchal systems.
For the past five thousand years his systems were put in place for the subversion of the only spiritual bridge for its own healthy development – *womanhood*. An almost entire exclusion of woman from any position of influence or the right to her own self-determination. Now and then we see token positions given to women, and in that sphere of action where there is bound to engage in a

battle of the sexes, whereby the woman is bound to stifle and sacrifice her femininity.

This is the cause of today's world crises, about to bring the ultimate downfall of nations. For each system was designed with one fatal error – that of not setting up itself to "see", that is, to perceive itself. For, it has suppressed its own transparency, – the high vantage point of delicate feminine perception, thus creating its own blindness.

Yet societies which have inherited this ruling-class pyramid can look at themselves in the social mirror if they choose. They only have to look at the present state of women and children. Today's women are so repressed they cannot break the cycle of their poverty and oppression to challenge the system effectively. Socialised to accept the status quo, woman has disarmed herself of the vigilance needed to affect any changes for herself and offspring, and passes this conditioning to the same oppressive male of tomorrow.

Any opposition by woman against such a condition is severely challenged. Self-effacement is still expected of her. She must remain inferior to men, for if they allow it otherwise, she will become a thorn in their side. Hence the ongoing saga of violence against women, insensitivity of government to the concerns of the vulnerable and the downtrodden.

Love – The Answer

With all the attacks upon the physical body today, especially the immune system, from inside as well as outside – the inner emotions as well as from psychic and environmental influences – the best, in fact, the only, remedy is to draw from the higher planes of love. That selfless love grounded only in the burning desire to serve humanity in the expression of our gifts and abilities, not to deceive. Uplifting creative activities can unite the different radiations within our being in the oneness of sheer power, *i.e.*, inner soundness.

Through the requisite exertion to align these energies within our being with love we finally become fiery flames, engulfing our weaknesses and defects of character and all obstacles that stand in our way, by transforming them into strength and nobility. Or, we may choose to continue along the sensual materialistic path of our self-indulgent passions towards the Darkness and succumb to the consequent autoimmune diseases, such osteoarthritis, cancer, AIDS *etc*.

In choosing to develop self-control, *i.e.*, learn to control our emotions (emanations), how we think, perceive, speak and act, as with a radio, we attune our own vibrations with the powerful healing and uplifting colour-radiations of the great Universe, perpetually pulsating downward.

Eventually the tapestry of our cloaks will attract that kind of attention like "Joseph's coat of many colours". We allow our intuitive perceptions, thoughts and actions to become beautifully coloured threads of radiation, reflecting that quality and harmonious tone as is determined by the strength of the colour combination in the threads we have chosen, *i.e.*, activities in which we engage in our daily lives.

With an understanding of the various bodies the human spirit wears for it to become active in the World of Matter, it is now clear that belonging to the spiritual, humans are not the earthly materialist he has become, but by nature is an *intuitive perceptive being.* Real life is ethereal-spiritual life, animating the gross physical body into an organism.

Organism is a function. In that the physical body – a gift from Nature – is given to us for the maturity of the spirit through activity, it is therefore the most important implement in the World of Matter. As the vehicle of the spirit, it is *the most precious possession* received for our entire lifetime, even if the body is diseased which, however, would perhaps not develop quickly had it been healthy. Disease and stress, or the disposition to them, are therefore signs that the physical body does not swing in harmony with the spiritual, thus cannot be supported and maintained.

It must be made clear, however, that because we bear spirit-seed within we do not automatically become human beings. We do not become human beings unless we allow the spirit as such to work within. In other words, learn to control oneself *correctly* – the temperament, the intellect which governs feelings and instincts, as in the urge for sex, food and other basic bodily requirements. So that over all we express from within, through words or direct action – our behavior is the exercise of complete control.

But how guilty are we of the sin of neglect of this most precious gift we have received? We rarely give the body the attention it requires until we have damaged it and caused pain and distress or until it prevents us from carrying out our daily activities, following some trifling pursuit or sport.

This is the basis for the misalignment of the energies of the body and spirit, creating what is called a "reverse-flow" phenomenon; that is, the directing of generative powers downward to the indulgence of our wrong attractions, to the point where our propensities become our weakness – psychically and physiologically – be it they draw attraction to the wrong kinds of foods, activities, lifestyles, or unhealthy surroundings. This is why we must begin the re-alignment where the breakdown has occurred – within the physical body.

The adolescent cycle is the beginning of this ruthless abuse. The frivolous and careless neglect and abuse of all kinds: for example, cultivating the intellect one-sidedly with subjects of study. Only to sustain such patterns with junk food, smoking, stimulants, excessive drinking, sleep deprivation – patterns which show up in adulthood as omissions which prevent the unfolding of talents and abilities for the fulfilment of *life's work and purpose.*

Only a strong, healthy body in normal physical condition can completely fulfil the purpose of one's existence. A body disturbed by this derangement upsets the absolutely necessary harmony between the body and spirit. Only a complete harmony brings about a healthy and strong inner development of the soul.

The care of the physical body is therefore of the most urgent necessity. We should give the healthy body all it needs if we expect to develop spiritually. We must observe it with all the care requisite for the proper activity of the most necessary implement. We cannot do too much in caring for it, keeping it pure and clean, because it is indispensable for our life span in the maturity of the spirit to self-consciousness. Due to its normal condition a healthy and unrestrained body will always harmonise with the spirit, thereby providing it with that necessary firm foundation for our moral development.

Invaluable, therefore, is the cycle of adolescence, since the endocrine glands are particularly involved with the blood-radiation and the passing of hormones into the bloodstream. Since this cycle marks the beginning of the unfolding of generative powers along with the *transformation of the blood*, parents, guardians and educators can only appreciate the value of guiding youths in showing them the importance of the proper development of the physical body, as the first order of self-discipline, even if they failed themselves in this respect. For only such enables the blood to form the right composition at every stage of our logical development.

To achieve this completeness, youths should be guided to understand why absolute harmony must prevail in the composition of the radiations of the physical body. This will provide the spirit with the best means of protection, development and advancement. It is for this reason, in addition to (1) maintaining that perfect equipoise between the intellectual (masculine) and intuitive (feminine) brains, attention is also given to (2) the right choice of foods and (3) correct breathing[12]. These three approaches will form matrix of energies to bring about a mental adjustment, if there is to be any progress in attaining the Unified Self.

Before we look at correct diet and breathing, we must first return to the point in the introduction where reference was made to dark or not-so-dark thoughts and desires and how the body attracts influences of similar nature which possess the body and afflict it with sickness and disease.The radiation of the spirit-part becomes greatly weakened by this ongoing tension. To this weakened spiritual-radiation is further added more physical trauma caused by ongoing irritation of cells through toxins. Toxins of intestinal origin are frequently found to be either a cause or contributing factor to many clinical phenomena.

This creates regulatory rigidity in the otherwise fluid flow-pattern of the substrate in the organism, restricting movement due to enzymatic reduction and oxygen deficiency. "Friendly" bacteria – which otherwise help support the organism – circulate in the blood, reproducing and generating infinite numbers of "bad" bacteria and parasites of different shapes and forms aimed at afflicting the host organism. All because of our repressed or dark emotions.

Toxic cells and faulty genetic dispositions, alter the cell's DNA and impairs its regulation which leads to disease. Cells no longer receive the right spiritual information from the autonomic nerve impulses for their development. They literally starve and disrupt mental function. It is difficult to fathom how disease develops, but they make themselves known at the onset by functional disturbances in many organs: headaches, high or low blood pressure, general malaise, lack of appetite or motivation, drab complexion, coated tongue, halitosis, wounds in the mouth, problems with skin, hair and nails, breast pathology, intestinal inflammation, food allergies, bloating, gastritis, illocecal valve incompetence, hiatal hernia, heartburn, hoarseness, catarrhs, ear noises, diarrhea, constipation, weight loss, lower back pain and sciatica, impaired sight and hearing, depression, senility, schizophrenia, epilepsy, weak concentration or poor memory, among others.

Toxicity and the Immune System

For more than forty years of intensive research in pleomorphism, symbiosis and cyclogeny of microorganisms, Professor Dr. Guenther Enderlein (1872-1968) of Germany, expanded his work upon the premise that all warm-blooded organisms house a primal *plant germ*, which is said to have invaded the entire range of mammal species millions of years ago. According to the French researcher A. Bechamp these plant-germ continue to live after the death of the organism that host them and out of which microorganisms can develop. Through environmental influences, these organisms can change form and develop to manifest as parasites.

This belies the allopathic medical view that there is only a single form and function of microorganisms, it does not recognise cyclic developmental. Hence the allopathic philosophy that "bad" microorganisms must be "fought" and "exorcised" with antibiotics; instead of the immune biological non-violent (pleomorphic) approach of regulation of their colony.

Aspergillus niger and *Mucor racemosus* are two species viewed as the cause for numerous illnesses. Aspergullus phases are said to appear relatively infrequently in their pathological forms *i.e.*, only in tuberculosis and paratuberculous disease; whereas Mucor symbiosis in its growth phases is much more involved in the development of pathogenic functions or changes. All human beings acquire this "embiont" via the placenta and house at least its primitive phases in cells and body fluids. With the exception of tuberculosis and syphilis, the multifaceted illnesses are said to be linked to the mucor parasite which attack mainly the mucosa block of the intestines.

Along with her defective genes, a mother-to-be also shares some of her immune protection with her developing fetus across the placenta in the form of antibodies (synthesised blood protein which develops in plasma cells to attack antigens, *e.g.* lymphocytes). Depending on her level of toxicity, she may send too many antibodies, or she may even transmit antigens circulating in her blood to the fetus. Hence some immune reactions begin in the baby's body even before birth. If after birth, the mother's breast milk, which is supposed to provide immunity to the child, carries antigenic material (be it bacteria, bacterial toxins, viruses, substances and toxins of animal and plant origin, foreign protein) to the baby, or if the child is not breast-fed long enough, its immunity suffers.

Intestinal toxemias are the most important primary and contributing causes of many disorders and diseases of the human body. The main sources of intestinal toxmia are functional disorders of the gastrointestinal tract such as hypo- or sub-acidity, infections and toxicity, as well as foreign antigens from specific components of foods. Intensive contact between foreign substances occurs in the inner wall of the intestines. This exposes the colon, the concentration of intestinal contents and intestinal flora to the largest number of antigens. It is for this reason the intestinal tract is richly supplied with immunological mechanisms: lymphocytes, plasma cells, macrophages (scavenger cells), plaques and mesentric lymph nodes, because it has to cope with a continuous influx of antigens.

Faulty diet or intestinal obstruction are the main causes of intestinal toxemia. Where there is a liver insufficiency the blood cannot be detoxified sufficiently, causing various toxins to be absorbed into the bloodstream. Toxins form chemical substances which poison as they enter the general circulation and exert deleterious effects before being excreted by the kidneys. The result of the intoxication is to produce a pathological change in the tissues, or to aggravate a previously existing condition.

Pathological change results from the development of an endobiont (apathological, low phase of the mucor parasite). Fibrin (a blood clot), is the endobiont's highest form, before the transformation of the parasistic germ from the primitive phase into the bacterial phase. The higher the level of fibrin in bloodstream, the greater the damage to blood vessels.

In its lower primitive or mutual phase, the microorganism is called a symbiont, which supports the body's metabolic activity in keeping the equilibrium in the flora system, especially the mucosa barrier against the entry of competing yeast antigens in the intestines, thus strengthening the defense. The higher the endobiont rises in its developmental three-phase series – virus (microbe), bacteria and fungus (the end which constitutes the starting point of its new cycle) the more toxic it becomes, giving rise to pathogenic (endobiontic) diseases and death. Over the course of the process, the endobiont usually causes tumor to develop.

Disease, however, does not mark the end of life, but indicate healing processes which attempt to return a disturbed symbiosis (the organism with its interdependent community of different symbionts) to the original healthy condition. Whether "self", the biological self-healing forces of the organism will win over the disease, or whether the symbiont is able to develop unchecked into a parasite, depend on the condition of the environment (the body fluids around the cells). If the environment is damaged through unhealthy nutrition and lifestyle, with their resultant disturbance of the acid-base equilibrium by environmental toxins, infection, depression, complaints of old age, *etc.*, the self is incapable of restoring its symbiotic equilibrium. The disease will damage the body.

Pathologist, Sean Moore at McMaster University has tried for nearly thirty years to convince his colleagues that cholesterol is not the primary cause of atherosclerosis, the hardening of the arteries. Though cholesterol worsen lesions and the accompanying plaque build-up, he believes the culprit could be a virus, an enzyme, a toxic byproduct of tobacco – even a hormone produced by unhappy childhood, injuring blood vessel walls and giving rise to tiny lesions. A hypothesis, light-years ahead the present rigid focus on "saturated fats", but left him without acknowledgement in scientific journals, because of present rigid beliefs.

His position is that atherosclerosis is the side-effect of a healing process. When tiny lesions form inside arteries, they attract platelets and other "healing" cells. This proliferation forms the tough, brittle substance, called plaque. As plaque accumulates, it becomes a regulatory blockage, *i.e.*, a blockage of circulating fluids in the body (a clot) which impedes the flow of oxygen through the blood. The slightest weakening of any tissue, any organ increases the valence (combining power) of the endobiont and further weakens the diseased organism. If the blockage is of the conorary artery, it can destroy the heart muscle by depriving it of oxygen lodged in other parts of the vessel.

This complex includes, among other things: connective tissue weakness, improper blood clotting, rheumatism, arthritis, spondylosis, tonsillitis, lymphotasis, diabetes, gout, tumors of all kinds, anemia, leukemia, cerebral sclerosis, paralysis,

The metabolism of a cancer sufferer diverges from normal metabolism. Cancer cells show exactly that of the form of a fungal organism in the individual, responsible for the fermentation and decomposition conditions. This led one Professor Enderlein to conclude the following: "cancer constitutes a fermentation and decomposition condition which is forced upon the host organism (whether human being or animal) by a parasitic fungus and its developmental forms."[13]

Toxicity and the Liver

Toxins not only cause the immune system to suffer, but poison the liver. The body's detoxification process is primarily the responsibility of the liver. Blood flowing from the stomach and intestines is not returned directly from these organs to the heart, but is conveyed by the portal vein to the liver. Once the portal vein has transported the blood to the liver, the vein divides like an artery and ultimately ends in capillary-like vessels (sinusoids). From these sinusoids, substances absorbed from the intestines become exposed to liver parenchymal cells. These cells hepatocyes, act upon such substances in many ways.

Ideally, hepatocytes protect the body by detoxifying it. But when there are too many toxins for the liver to act upon, it burdens the body with chronic intoxicating symptoms. Mucosal injury, especially when absorption of toxic substance takes place faster than the liver can detoxify, and toxemia lead to death.

Phenol and skatole are two poisons which escape liver action and adversely affect the brain. Because the brain is chemically based, these toxins only serve to alter it's chemistry. Tryptophan, the amino acid which yields serotonin – the brain's "mellow chemical" which keeps us cool, calm and collected – produces skatole and indole when digestion is impaired. These chemicals give feces its unpleasant odor. Such malodorous compounds agitate and disturb the brain, because their abnormal functions produce substances such as octopamine which are called "false neurotransmitters". They replace the normal transmitters, whose job it is to accurately transfer messages across the brain, leaving the consciousness further scattered, unable to properly monitor or maintain the organism's immune defenses. Other endobiontic toxic substances produced in the large intestines which have a negative influence on hepatic (liver) metabolism, include amines, phenols and histamine, the result of putrefied proteins.

So one can see why smoking, with its carbon dioxide poisoning, invariably shatters the nerves and overworks the liver. "Quite apart from the smokers themselves, having to breathe in such tobacco smoke which hampers the normal development of many an organ in infants and children, especially the necessary firmness and strengthening of the liver, which is particularly important for every person, because the functioning in the right and healthy manner it can prevent the establishment of a cancerous centre as the surest and best means of resistance of this plague" (Abd-ru-shin).

Toxins, Liver and the Emotions

Just as intestinal toxemia caused from improper digestion can disturb the consciousness and agitate the emotions, disturbed emotions weaken digestion and create intestinal toxemia, exciting the immune system to react against the toxin until immunity collapses altogether. Why? Human character is influenced by the limbic system – the complex system of nerve pathways and networks in the brain – involved in the expression of instinct and mood activities in the endocrine and motor systems of the body. This centre for the endocrine and motor regulation is placed directly above the hypothalamus and influences the emotional reaction of a person and thereupon its psychic-affective total behavior. Hence the major influence on the mental origin (psychogenia) of many diseases, *e.g.*, diseases of the digestive system, particularly the stomach.

This is the link between criminal behavior and brain toxicity, which again leads back to impaired liver function. All processes in the liver are of central importance for the organism. Metemperically, the liver represents "good sense" and sanity, so when overstrained, it cannot totally neutralise contaminants. It then becomes the seat of fear and it brings about anger and rage which develop the urge for other sensory indulgences. A condition which should be looked out for in early childhood to help balance and normalise the organism.

Iris analysis according to Flink, shows this "disharmony line": horizontal signs of a non-specific type (lacunae, broken rays, dark areas) from 3 o'clock to 9 o'clock, especially in the left iris. Symptomatically, this is accompanied by a full range of liver disturbances, hepato-renal syndrome and liver-heart-kidney syndrome, to name a few. He found that, "the individual is always annoyed with him/herself and others." This forms the basis for one's inner dichotomy or vice-versa - the inability to perform conscious liberated actions.

The liver, therefore, warrants recognition, not only the most important organ to target for research into criminal behavior but also cancer-resistance. It is widely accepted, at least in complimentary medicine that cancerous growth is conditioned by the incapacity and insufficient activity of the liver".

METABOLIC CLEANSE

In summing up the above processes, we can say that in some way or other we all inherit susceptibility to particular diseases. However, we may not experience symptoms or may notice only small alterations in body functions, because the body addresses this disposition in – the "robbing Peter to pay Paul" style. When the body's ability to compensate is exhausted, pathological developments produce symptoms – the pre-cancerous stage of disease. If the process continues uncorrected, in most cases the altered body function causes irreversible structural damage to tissues.

What could be more effective in correcting alterations to normal body chemistry than by natural means? In the Law of Attraction of Homogeneous Species, biological treatment is most likely to help sufferers – that is, if the degenerative process has not already made recovery impossible, and even so, it can prolong life and freedom from pain. Chemical treatment hardly results in cure, this we know from the increasing number of illnesses. Whole food complexes have been clinically proven to have that same drug-like effect on the body, because they restore normal blood-composition which fortifies the spirit, granting the opportunity for the indwelling volition to unfold its personal power.

Again, the success of any biological approach depends on the existing toxic condition of the organism. Research confirms that in all precancerous phases, one finds higher valenced endobionts (parasites) in the blood. If the blood is the life of the body, as discussed later, what fraction of life are we living if its composition is so gravely altered.

Therefore, alongside a full scope of abundant and free natural movements of the physical body and good hygienic conditions of life regarding, in particular, one's sleeping area, the hygiene of the internal organs is the critical factor which contributes to health and longeviety. All three factors combine to maintain to an optimum muscle tone, not gym equipment or cosmetic surgery.

Internal hygiene forms the basis for the efficient absorption of nutrients for the body to utilise. From time to time, especially during spring and summer's abundance of fruits and vegetables, special remedies should be used to stimulate the body's detoxification process. Pathological changes, however, may necessitate detoxifying and supporting all organs and systems of the body with natural remedies to eliminate the digested toxins through the urinary tract, colon, skin and lungs. Hence the following organs and systems must be taken into consideration in the detoxification process.

Immune System

The immune system operates as the body's security force, up to the highest level of operation in its connection to the aura. Its maximum protection of our physical, mental, emotional, social environments is measured on how alert and swift it is in its execution to stress factors. Intestinal parasitic microbes can impair the immune system, weakening our psychic and physical defense, which give rise to physical as well as mental ill-health. In that eighty percent of the immune system lies in the gut and eliminatory canal, one cannot overemphasise with what urgency we must see to the reduction of these microbes, first by intake of biological remedies for secretion and then by reestablishing normal intestinal flora by administering intestinal symbionts, *e.g.*, lactobacillus acidophilus or lactobacillus bifidus, as well as calcium ascorbate and trace minerals.

Lymphatic System

The lymphatic system is a pathway of vessels running through the body play a major role in the body's defense mechanisms. It is also the body's transport system, which is most active within the millions of tiny villi in the inner surface of the intestines, "sucking" up small digested food particles, thus dramatically increasing the surface area of the small intestines. Its importance also lies in its distribution of fluid and nutrients throughout the body; it ensures that excess fluid and proteins are drained off so that the tissues do not swell. In addition, it makes sure that substances like fats, cell debris, foreign bodies, bacteria and products of metabolism are carried away. In the process, however, toxins may enter the lymphatic system and be deposited in the interstitial connective tissue. Intestinal bacteria especially, increases active and passive absorption of antigens (potentially dangerous foreign substances) and may therefore cause excessive strain on the gut.

Heart

The heart is one circulatory organ, without which the lungs cannot function, and vice versa. They are called co-workers at the very head of life and all its energies. If the heart is in poor health, then the prognosis for healing is poor. The cardiovascular system must be intact as a requisite for adequate renal function; which if is insufficient causes dyskinesia (back-up of the liver and bile duct), leading to poor digestion and absorption of essential vitamins and minerals.

Kidneys

The renal system is the major means by which the body rids itself of poisons and toxins. Once the toxins are in the bloodstream the kidneys are the only filters left that can de-activate them. If the renal system is not well suited for the task, it may become irritated, the kidneys, urethra and bladder infected. Interference with the kidneys' normal functions such as regulation of fluids and minerals results in fluid retention and/or mineral deficiencies, and possibly crystalization of minerals into stones.

Liver

Known as the organ of equilibrium, in a psychic and a physical sense, its over 500 physical functions involve regulating and supporting the work of all the other organs and systems, especially in its round-the-clock detoxification of nutrients for the body's blood supply. It is said that the difference between an individual with disease symptoms and one without is often related to whether or not the liver can handle intestinal toxins and still have the capacity to do other jobs.

Pancreas

The pancreas is called the cleanup hitter of the digestive system. What the mouth and the stomach fails to digest, the pancreas calls in enzymes along with alkaline bile from the liver and the gall bladder to finish. One of its most important function, however, is to secrete the enzyme insulin, to allow the body to balance the sugar levels in the blood. This remains one of the most grievously damaged organs of the body, because of overwork from high dietary intakes of sugar[14] . In addition, not chewing carbohydrates stresses the pancreas further due to the reliance on digestive enzymes for digestion. Therefore, greater importance is placed on the detoxifying function of the pancreas, in an enzymatic and immunological sense.

ENZYME THERAPY

Enzyme comes from the Greek word *inleaver*, en (in) + zyme (leaver). Enzymes are basically RNA (ribonucleic acid), one of the two organic acids acting as a catalyst in every nucleus and cytoplasm of cells responsible for formation of proteins, the main constituents of cell membranes. The other organic acid, DNA, (deoxyribonucleic acid), is responsible for the overall function of the cell.

All living things contain enzymes, without which they could never live. Enzymatic activity is responsible for every biochemical reaction occuring in living matter. They increase reaction rates, regulate substrates, products and themselves, fight entropy, have intelligence and maintain energy; gait reaction accelerates and decelerates them. However, in that they are biologically alive they can be exhausted and become deficient in the human body. According to Dr. Edward Howell, the pioneer of "Enzyme Nutrition", when we eat cooked enzyme deficient food, the body is forced to produce enzymes needed for digestion. This stealing of the enzymes from other parts of the body compensates for enzymes along various organ systems and tissues of the body. The resulting metabolic dislocations may be the direct cause of many chronic incurable diseases.

Nature's plan, however, was for food enzymes to help with digestion instead of requiring the body's digestive enzymes to carry the whole burden. Hence a diet high in raw, organic and adulterated foods as the ideal choice. This would place much less demand on the body to manufacture and secrete digestive enzymes, so as to expend more energy in manufacturing the thousands of metabolic enzymes it needs to run the entire body. But with today's modern living we have long diverted from this natural eating pattern and are thus left with bodies which can no longer resist pathological damage. Hence enzyme therapy, the ingestion of prepared whole food concentrates combined with the concentrated plant and microbal enzymes needed to balance altered body physiology.

Three dimensional, that is, bearing physical, chemical, and electrical properties, enzymes are to the human body what the elemental forces (of fire, water, air and earth) are to the foundation of Nature. Enzymes like to work in groups, supporting each other, binding and releasing, synthesising and displacing manner, constantly changing the blood radiation to bring about a harmonious body and mind relationship based on the right choice of nutrients.

There are three categories of enzymes: (1) food enzymes, which are contained in all raw food and start digestion in the cardiac portion of the stomach; (2) digestive (pancreatic) enzymes, which are secreted by the body to digest our foods; and (3) metabolic enzymes, by which all our organs and tissues are run – structuring protein, fats and carbohydrates and keeping our biological clocks ticking synchronistically – our breathing, thinking, talking, moving and our immunity.

When there is a depletion of the body's supply of enzymes to carry out its functions – due to drugs, radiation, toxins, poor eating and lifestyle habits, functional disorders of the gastrointestinal tract, severe intestinal infections, bacteria toxins and others – disharmony (dis-ease) results. This disrupts our biological clock's rhythm and damage DNA.

Symptoms of enzyme deficiency are fatigue and energy loss, poor digestion, inflammation, endocrine (hormone) imbalance, toxic syndrome, weakness, pain, premature ageing. Physiologically, it leads to pathological enlargement of the pituitary gland, pancreas and liver, and decreased digestive capacity, assimilation of nutrients and elimination of toxins. A substitution of plant source enzymes to predigest foods, with the correct choice of nutrition, optimises digestion, absorption, and assimilation of foods to help the body repair itself and reset the biological clock for harmonious functioning.

THE LAW OF NUTRITION

In that reconditioning the body uses correct nutrients as the means to bring about harmonious function, great emphasis is placed on the proper digestion, absorption and utilisation of nutrients. Eating the correct food stimulates certain metabolic changes through the body fluids which act on the different systems, such as glandular, circulatory, nervous, excretory, *etc.*, and bring complete change in the personality.

Though choosing the right foods on its own will not harmonise body and mind, any activity that has the organising power of Natural Law brings the favor of Natural Law with it. Observing the Natural Laws with respect to nutrition provides the healthy soil for full activity. Violation of these laws transgresses the Laws of Creation and only disease can ensue. If we do not observe all the health laws with scrupulous fidelity, relying more on Nature and less on medicines and special remedies, and remitting no efforts and sparing no exertion to restore digestion, then we can only half think, study, remember, feel, transact business, or do or enjoy anything.

"You are what you eat", therefore stands as law. We set dietary patterns based on what makes us feel good, and we repeat these patterns day after day. Each basic food component, protein, fat, sugar and starch, influences the body temperament, driving the endocrine system in a predictable manner. This choice, however, has a lot to do with genetic hereditary conditions as well as our spiritual maturity, choices which contribute to the quality of the blood composition. Neurophysiologists, specifically Abravenal's success in body-type programming, have established that our food cravings, what smells and tastes good and what does not, are affected by the hypothalamus gland which monitors the body fluids, influences our taste buds and sense of smell, and drives the endocrine system via the pituitary gland. Such conscious choices begin at puberty, when spirit unites with the material body.

In that the digestion of food and drink subserve intellect and moral sentiment - converted into thought and emotion, different kinds of food are bound to produce different mental and moral traits. Would not, therefore biologically wholesome foods grown in organic conditions yield the most life-force? Whereas heavy, rich devitalised foods sap it, especially from our immune defense system, the brain and the spiritual bodies? Emphasis must be placed on a wholesome moderate diet, that is, foods as close to their natural state as possible. This refines the perceptions, cultivating the favorable blood-composition suited to our respective talents, and at the correct time in our temperamental life-cycles.

In addition to artificial chemical and pesticides added to our food, there must be great concern for the aggressive lobbying to legitimise hybridisation and genetic engineering of foods, a practice which will only be catastrophic to the human body. For whereas chemical fertilisers alter the natural enzymes in foods, genetic engineering breaks down the genetic fundamental barriers and permanently changes the genetic code of plants and animals by combining the genes of completely unrelated species into "new" species and not in accord with the Natural Laws of logical development.

What remains is hybrid offspring, void of the essential nutrients in the required amount and of the superior quality Nature stipulated to be so. Vegetables and fruits are genetically engineered to reduce farming and transportation costs and extend shelf-life indefinitely without losing the appearance of freshness; fish, poultry, and livestock are crossed and fed to yield more quickly and abundantly.

The consequences of such greed and arrogance can only lead to dire health implications for the countries which practice such methods. And like Adam in shifting the blame to Eve said: "Lord the woman you gave me as mate, she gave me of the tree, and I did eat", so do we support such industries in gulping down those hamburgers – or not caring if our children do – from mass-produced, assembly-line livestock to using harmful chemicals to clean our homes, while still grieving the cruelty of those who destroy the rain forest and pollute the oceans with their greed and irreverence to Nature, as documentaries show.

A recent Canadian study shows childhood asthma cases have risen dramatically from 2.5 percent in 1978-9 to 11.2 percent in 1994-5, with cancer and immune diseases also increasing at alarming rates. And this is only the tip of the iceberg, for after a prolonged period of trying to digest all these alien substances, the body's enzyme supply will eventually deplete, and the lymphatic system become exhausted. And for any form of healing to take place we must again return to Nature, which alone furnishes the organisms requisite for executing her respective functions for the working of the animistic faculties, which are implements of the spiritual.

To be natural and nature are one, the unadulterated effects of animistic activity. Nature must remain what it is, that which is able to be formed and to unite its basic species, that is, must remain unchanged by human hands. Only in the way that Nature, with its animistic workings produce unions is there found support for developing power radiations from unite homogenous species, with lasting effects. Unions which do not precisely accord with Natural Laws form radiations which harm one another, bringing catastrophic consequences.

But just the thought of such an ideal, natural diet can seem overwhelming as can the millions of books and tapes on the market, all claiming to offer the right knowledge. What is even more fundamental, however, is just as there are the different races of humans, within these homogenous groupings are different blood or constitution types. What direction is safer then, than following that as is observed in Nature?

Native Foods and Their Seasons

If we learn to observe the workings of nature we cannot help but adapt ourselves accordingly. First we will realise that foods produced in the region where we are born gives us more vitality. This happens, because the physical body is connected with that zone of the earth; connected with all the stars of the particular region and with the radiations present there. Hence, only that place where we are born can give our bodies exactly what it needs for health and longevity.

Nature provides these foods, zone by zone, always in the right season and perfectly balanced with the requisite nutrients for the body of one born there. These foods should only be eaten at those times the earth naturally produces them, not as fast as hot-house or genetic manipulation can produce them. It follows, therefore, that only within these seasons does their nourishment support the building of the body. For what other reason would nature be so systematic in her reproduction? We do not just celebrate our birthday when we feel like it. Why, then, would we grow and eat foods out of the season that Nature dictates?

And if we should only eat these foods in the seasons they are provided, it means that the body only needs these foods at the correct time the zone provides them, since humans and our surroundings are intimately connected. Nature offers continuous change in the foods just as the body really needs them, and in the proper sequence – apples in apple season, berries in berry season. If the soil in which fruits are grown is rich and organic, the fruits are so nutritious and full of sweet-flavored strength that only a few are needed to satisfy the body. So also are herbs, which are only beneficial at times when they are in full vigour and bloom, suited for the building and maintenance of a healthy body.

Migration

Those of us who have migrated may ask, how may we obtain the requisite nourishment while living away from the land of our birth? This the slave-drivers discovered only too well in the Caribbean and the Americas when their "bounty" died as fast as they arrived. Not until their native foods were finally transported along with the people and grown in these new regions, did the average life-span of the captives began to average twenty-seven years.

Immigrants to new lands with different climatic zones find at first, that only when they eat imports from their native lands do they feel vigorous, and a trip back home every now and then the greatest medicine. But after a while they notice a change in the body's need for its indigenous nourishment. A psychic adjustment allows for the radiation of their bodies to adapt to the radiation of the new surrounding. Slowly the personality alters; together with the light and air, they absorb the requisites for life on that soil, and must likewise adopt the food natural to that country. They acclimatise. Their blood changes, and the radiation of their blood facilitates connection with the new zone.

Hence migration to a colder climate would require the consumption of more grains and meats, especially during winter; whereas the strong fats and the smoked foods of the far north is no longer needed for one who has migrated to temperate zones. Those in the torrid zones require less meat and more fruits and vegetables, in order to cool one's temperament.

So to this concern, the answer is that the right harmony must be found in the middle-way. At first there must be a careful balancing so that the basis of the nutrition comes from foods imported from our zone of origin. With proper care, a bridge can be constructed which, for a time, makes it possible to unfold their full powers, though not permanently. Every now and then they must return to the land of their birth, in order to obtain new vitality, though this will never offer a long healthy life-span. Such only comes about when one's spirit is allowed to unfold on its soil of origin.

It is not arbitrary or accidental that we come in different forms and colours. The different races and peoples came about as the nations and peoples migrated and settled in different zones from the equator; and accordingly, Nature fashioned the different bodies and shapes to accompany and indicate the same traits of character, and, at the same time, the different foods for our nourishment and maintenance. Every distinct human form and colour indicates some particular proclivity or passion. This is the law of genetics – the DNA blueprint we carry within us and which has been replicated within us continuously through the blood in our ancestral lineage.

The genetic memory lies within every animal, every plant; in fact, every branch of natural History furnishes infinite proof of this principle. Every kind of fish, fowl, and creeping thing, from the beginning of time, always kept, and will keep, its own specific form, to which each individual of every class, genius, and species conforms – except where cross breeding and intermixing occurs. In the case of humans, the effects of racial interbreeding not only cause character defects, torn intuitive perceptions, sickness and even sterility, but also a degeneration, uprooting, and the final ruin of entire indigenous tribes and peoples, because the basis for natural growth was eroded.

This law of conformity is what is required to achieve body alignment; a readjustment whereby foods are carefully selected to strengthen or weaken, even displace certain blood radiations, so that the temperament harmonise not only with our natural environment, but with the world-at-large, the entire Universe.

It requires care, however, to ensure that this readjustment does not happen so suddenly, it disturbs the physical body. A derangement would then upset the necessary harmony between the physical body and the spirit, which leads to the possibility of eccentricities. Any new or different approaches should be gradual. Rapidity in any transition causes a weakening; in this case, the physical body suffers, even if it still appears to be in good health. A body weakened in this manner is never able to regain vigour.

VEGETARIANISM

Other than regular and extensive fasts, imposing privation upon the body which weakens it and renders it unfit for the fulfilment of *life's work and purpose*, vegetarianism is another radical transition. Though noble in its attempt to correct the radically deficient manner of eating today, the necessary transition is usually lacking. Although proven to refine the nervous system and regenerate the human physiology, ennobling it, strengthening it and helping it to good recovery, adopting vegetarianism as permanent way of life can only be supported in its entirety by nature in the next stage in the evolution of human development.

That era dawns, yes, but only when it sets in and with it the collective refinement of human minds, will the physical body also change its form to a higher species of matter in which the animal passions are no longer dominant, and with it different food selections as Nature sees fit for its support. That will be the stage of a more advanced human-spiritual maturity, when the hearth of the volition and thoughts of people become pure, and in such a way that life becomes peaceful.

Then will radiation of our blood no longer carry that primitive gene and its predominant element which requires eating flesh to feed the passions and urges of the physical body. Until then, meat remains the grounding element for our physical bodies as determined by our present collective level of consciousness.

Hence, in the continuous "cycle of life", animals will no longer need to give themselves up to sustain humans at the top of the food chain. What animal activists call cruelty to animals pertaining to do with our diet is, today, a survival of the human species. They only have to look within every apple to see that therein slumbers the capacity for it to enrich life with new apple trees, with flowers and fruit. It is the automatic course of the Primordial Laws of Creation which endowed the apple with that capacity, and which forces it to act as it does in order to fulfil its task in Creation. It always and inevitably fulfils one task. So is it with every beast of prey. Every species of life in Nature serves as a part of the food chain of another and, has the built-in instinct to preserve its species or face extinction. Nothing in this Creation is without a task. Even in death and decay there is still movement, value and gain.

Vegetarianism is good when used temporarily. It can even be practised for years at a time in the case of sick people; for it helps to alleviate some disorders, assist in one-sidedly strengthening of some physical organ by which the spirit is further uplifted. Such is the case with cancer and other autoimmune diseases linked to toxemia of parasistic origin. Parasites grow by passing through various intermediate stages to become bacteria by greedily devouring ingested proteins, especially co-created through improper nutrition. Hence the restriction of a high protein, acidic diet – particularly meat, fish and eggs, is advised to curtail their growth and return them to their lower (non-pathogenic) alkaline microbal-form.

Along with biological remedies, lacto-vegetarianism is advised, because it reestablishes the acid-base equilibrium and may prevent and cure illnesses; it improves the general function of organs; and leads to the psychological and spiritual constitution of renewed well-being. But it should not be lasting. If the body is to maintain its full vigour, after recovery, one must gradually return to the diet to which he or she is accustomed. The appearance of well-being a vegetarian diet gives is only a deception. It is the result of the change, and all change is refreshing, even for the spirit.

One who suddenly deprives their body of the food of its genetic coding on a permanent basis, will notice it actually becomes weaker and weaker and sensitive to almost everything. Although there appears to be attributes of composure and equanimity, they also experience diminution of strength. This definite kind of weakness shows itself to be agreeable with nothing, and depressing, because it does not originate from any disease.

The equanimity it gives, however, comes like healthy old age where only the body weakens; until suddenly it cannot produce the generative power the spirit needs to fully accomplish *life's work and purpose.*

When the harmony of the body and spirit is disturbed, the power of the penetrating radiation of generative power is drawn off in the wrong direction – toward ongoing health concerns.

Vegetarianism And The Sexual Urge

What most vegetarians notice is a slight abatement of their sexual urge, which is at times applauded as progress. But this does not mean that the spirit is ennobled through vegetarian diet. It only means that generative powers, which also fuel sexual instinct, have been lowered, without which one cannot achieve normal development; for the capacity for spiritual surging is lessened. And this can lead to eccentric lifestyles.

Yes, we should never allow ourselves to be mastered by the sexual impulses, nor become slaves to our instincts. But a lowering in this manner is not to be applauded, because it is the result of a one-sided and abnormal cultivation.

We do not need deprivation of what is good for us. We should stand above our sexual instinct, that is, not force incontinence upon ourselves. With pure inner morality, we practice self-control so that we do no harm to ourselves and subsequently to others.

The moderation of the sexual instinct is by no means to be dependent on the lessening of generative power. Quite to the contrary, generative power advances the human spirit, liberates it from its dependence on the coarser sexual instinct, and remains the best means to accomplish this.

And let us not kid ourselves; sexual instinct has its purpose. It is the result of the radiation animistic emanations interacting upon matter (the physical body) through the nervous system, giving it warmth and movement for the requisite renewal, advancement and development of matter – procreation. It is the most beautiful gift given to the human spirit. This is why it is called having nature, an act in which we should engage in as if paying tribute to Nature. According to Harberehl, professor at the Sexology Institute in Hamburg: "During sexual intercourse, our bodies manufacture a powerful hormone cocktail that has an immensely positive impact." In short, as long as sex is not unnatural or excessive, it makes us happier, healthier and wiser. So to toy with one's healthy demand for sexual intercourse is like depriving it of fresh air, food and water and can only do more harm than good.

Meat and the Sexual Urge

The heavy consumption of meat aggravates the sexual instinct, thus sapping generative power. It is proven that a diet which is exclusively red meat, as is required for sports such as boxing to increase ferocity, can only produce the brutish behavior of the lion, tiger, shark, eagle, *etc.*, whose diet is the same.

Therefore, the most sensible approach is the middle-way. There must be a careful balanced diet in the necessary intake of protein, based on the individual's own requirement. A moderate approach would restrict the diet to white meat such as: poultry, veal, deer, sheep, which by their docile nature, can only bring about the same in the temperament.

Such should be balanced with cereals and an increased amount of vegetables, which keep the system cool, promote mental quietness, intellectual clearness, and moral elevation. Non-enzyme inhibitor, cruciferous (pungent) vegetables such as bok choy, broccoli (cooked), kale, rutabaga, and turnips are found to support liver detoxification pathways. With less meat and more vegetables, grains, and fruits, we become less sensual, and more creative and pure at heart.

Protein is needed to build and repair tissue such as muscles, blood, bone, skin and internal organs. It is the main constituent of all the cell membranes. Dietary protein is needed to bind with free calcium in the blood for the utilisation of the latter by the structural tissue and the nervous system. In a healthy nervous system, protein and calcium are integrally involved in the release of neurotransmitters which propagate transmission of nerve impulses. When extracellular levels of proteins and calcium are low, irregular nervous reactions or anxiety can result.

Protease is the digestive enzyme which breaks down protein into essential amino acids, of which as much as 56 percent are converted by the liver into glucose for use in energy metabolism, hence a major source of energy for the brain and cells. Eight essential amino acids are needed to maintain health in humans: leucine, isoleucine, lysine, methionine, phenylalanine, theonine, tryptophan, and valine. If these amino acids are not present at the same time and in the definite proportion, the other amino acids, in whole and in part, cannot be used for protein metabolism. All of these essential amino acids are available in proteins produced in the seeds of plants, but because plant sources are often weak in lysine and tryptophan, nutrition experts advise supplementing the diet with animal protein from meat, eggs, and milk, which contain all the essential acids.

Protease deficiency has been clinically observed, not only to lead to a loss of desire for meat (a built-in mechanism of the hypothalamus to turn off the taste in one who intolerant to or cannot digest this particular food group), but also sexual indifference. For due to the body's inability to digest and assimilate protein, this affects the supply of protein hormones (protease) which feeds the pituitary gland. One who is protein intolerant, *i.e.*, deficient in protease, finds meat and high-protein foods disagreeable. This is what has led many to become vegetarian – an unhealthy choice for the blood radiation.

Symptoms of protease deficiency can be any of the following: poor appetite; sense of fullness; depression; muscular weakness; lack of vigour and stamina; flabbiness of flesh; fluid retention; hair loss; poor resistance to and recovery from illness; impaired healing of wounds, among others. The result of a protease deficiency is that protein-based foods are poorly digested, which increases intestinal toxemia.

Meat remains the main source of protein for the human body. A diet containing meat is invaluable in maintaining the correct acidity of the blood serum, otherwise called, Extra Cellular Fluid (ECF), and bring about homeostasis of the blood alkaline/acid balance. More critical in preventing the above symptoms described, in addition to ensuring the harmonious relation of the sympathetic and parasympathetic branches of the nerves[15] , is a healthy lymphatic and cardiovascular system.

When there is a deficiency in protein, either through inadequate intake or poor digestion, the body craves simple sugars, known as the "sugar fix", leading many to consume far beyond the capacity the pancreas can handle, to fill this requirement, and to which our bodies eventually become intolerant. Then one experiences anything from hypoglycemia (seizure in extreme cases); respiratory problems (sinusitis, asthma); underactive thyroid (hypothyroidism); constipation or diarrhea, Candida albicans; mental and emotional problems including depression, mood swings, angry, aggressive, or violent behavior, anxiety attacks,, manic depression (bipolar disorders); hyperactivity/attention deficit disorder, among others.

Though an advocate of vegetarianism himself, an excerpt from Fowler's work confirms that the health and combined action of the organs has a great impact on character, particularly in directing it:

> "Health consists in the normal and vigorous exercise of all the physical functions, and disease in their abnormal action. Health is pleasurable, disease painful. Health is life, for life consists in the normal action of those same functions in which health consists. And to improve health is to increase life itself, and all its pleasures. Some writer has appropriately defined health thus:
>
> Planting your foot upon the green sward, looking around, and yielding yourself to whatever feelings naturally arise, health is proportionate to that buoyant, jubilant, exhilarating, ecstatic feeling which supervenes. It is to all our function what motive power is to machinery - sets them off with a rush and a bound. It both makes us happy, and causes everything else to increase that happiness.

But disease renders us miserable, and turns everything around us into occasions of misery. It both weakens and perverts our mental being. Indeed, health is the quintessence of every good - disease of every terrestrial evil. Poor indeed is he, however rich in money, in honors, in office, in everything else whatsoever, whose health is poor; for how can he enjoy his dollars and his honors? But rich indeed is he who is healthy, however poor in money, for he enjoys whatsoever he has and is. A rich man may, indeed, purchase a luxuriant dinner, but without health does not, cannot relish it; whereas a poor man with health, enjoys even a dry crust.

The rich need health to enjoy their riches; the poor doubly, in order to prevent becoming poorer. But to be poor and sickly is the uttermost of human evil. Nor can the poor afford to be sick; for their health is their all, to themselves and their families. Nor should they allow any thing whatsoever to impair it, but make health paramount.

Even the very talents of men depend mainly on health. Is not the brain confessedly the organ of the mind? Now, what means it, that the brain is the organ of the mind, but that all its conditions similarly affect the mentality? And since the states of the body and brain act reciprocally - consequent of that vast network of nerves which ramify throughout every part and parcel of the body, and terminate in the brain - of course all existing conditions of the body similarly affect these nerves, and thereby the brain, and therefore the mind, rendering all the states of either body or mind reciprocal with those of the other. If the body is sick, or weak, or exhausted, or inflamed, or sleepy, or exhilarated, is not the mind equally so? Then to originate great thoughts, or to conceive pure and exalted sentiments, must not the brain be in a vigorous state? And in order to acquire cerebral vigor, must not all the bodily functions be equally vigorous? And to this end, must not those health-laws which cause the vigor be observed? Of what avail the learning of the sickly scholar, the talents of the invalid, or the goodness of the pious dyspeptic? They can do nothing, can enjoy nothing - are burdens to themselves and friends. Can we think, or remember, or study without that energy furnished by the body? No more than move machinery without motive power. How, then, can that boy become a great or learned man without possessing physical vigor? Or that delicate and beautiful girl a capable or good woman, wife, or mother without possessing animal vigor? Let it be forever and everywhere remembered, that both judgement and memory, reason and poetry, eloquence and philosophy, even morality and religion, all the virtues and all the vices - in short, one and all of the human functions, are all carried forward by animal power. Even the very sensual pleasures of the debauchee are exercises by this very animal force, and grow weak when and because it declines. And the physical power depends on the observance of certain physical laws, the violation of which weakens both body and mind, of course the first duty of every human being to himself and Creator - of parents to their children, of ministers to people, writer to reader, and one to all - is to -

LEARN TO OBEY THE HEALTH LAWS

And on this point is just where our whole educational system - collegiate especially - is radically defective. It eclipses more genius by weakening the body than it eliminates by study. Children are always smarter and better relatively than adults, because injured by that false educational system which impairs mind, memory, and morals by breaking down good physical constitutions. The Romans appropriately named their schools "gymnasia" from the muscular exercises which both formed their leading feature, and secured a strong mind, by strengthening the body. Our schools and colleges are, and will continue to be, fundamentally defective, till remodeled upon the basis of health as a means of scholarship and talents.

Nor intellect merely, but our very morals and piety, depend on health. Can we even pray or worship without vitality? And what is more, the very vices of mankind are consequent mainly on the infringement of the physical laws.

Hereditary conditions in parents cause a depravity in their children; yet even they do it by deranging their body. It is what men eat and drink, it is how they live sleep, *etc.*, it is their physiological conditions and habits, that cause nine-tenths of human depravity. Are not both children and adults depraved when cross, and cross because sick; that is, rendered sinful and unwell? Who does not know that drunkenness engenders depravity - makes the best men bad? But why, and how? By disordering the body. And since by alcohol, why not by tobacco, gluttony, and every other wrong physical state? Are not drunkenness and debauchery concomitants? Are not dyspeptics always irritable? The truth is, that all abnormal physical action causes abnormal mental action, which is sin. To become good and answer the end of their being, men must live right, must learn to eat right, and sleep, exercise, bathe, breathe, *etc.*, in accordance with nature's requisition. And nine-tenths of the sinfulness of mankind has this purely physical origin, and can be cured by physical means.

Health is the natural state of man, animal, vegetable, all that lives - is the ultimate of life. Like all else in nature, it has its laws; and these laws obeyed, will render it perfect from birth to death. It even requires immense violation of these laws seriously to impair it. Bird and beast are rarely unhealthy, except when rendered sickly by man. Has our benevolent Creator granted this greatest of boons to beasts, but denied it to man? No. None need ever be sick, for there are health laws, which, if obeyed, guarantee the very perfection of health. To become sickly is foolish; for it cuts off every pleasure, and induces every ill - is even wicked, for it is consequent only on a violation of the laws of our being, and all violation of law is sin. And the health laws are as much laws of God - written by his finger on our very constitution - as the Decalogue [Ten Commandments]. In short, none have any right to be sick. It is alike the privilege, as it as the sacred duty of one and all to be and keep well; that is, to observe the health laws. And to parents to keep their children well.

NATURAL MEDICINE IN CENSORSHIP

The question is asked, why the theory of intestinal toximia has not been discussed in recent times and why it is not well known today in the medical community? The abandonment of this idea over the years by the medical profession is said not to be based on any new scientific research proving error in the theory of intestinal toxemia. It is like certain ideas which fall into and out of favor as the years pass – regardless of their validity. The same is said of chiropractic therapy which, despite its great clinical usefulness, has been repeatedly "discovered" then abandoned or forgotten since ancient times. It was D.D. Palmer who revived this old healing and brought it to our attention."

But who needs scientific research or its endorsement when proven empirical methods (which should in no way be replaced by objective approaches) conclude that nutrition plays such critical role in the normal development of the physiology, and toxicity creates an impairment. Rather than adopting, where possible, the nutritional approach of those "called" to help humanity on this critical path – through the subjective methods derived from their clinical experience, *i.e.*, repeated observation and applications of methods to help the body to heal itself – doctors prefer to surgically remove all defected parts.

It is commonly held that all illnesses have a pre-degenerative phase, where there appears symptoms but no findings, *e.g.*, an abnormal glucose tolerance test after stress. It is this phase of the pathological process which leads to a diseased organ, and where preventative measures should be taken to reverse or halt its course, instead of suppressing damaged organs and tissue systems necessitating surgical removal.

It has being scientifically proven that genetic dispositions are best corrected with preventative treatments (phytotheraphy, homeopathy, enzyme therapy, *etc.,*) in children and young adults, to slow or stop the course of an illness. This is not to say that regeneration in not possible in one's later years by stimulating the body's power of resistance and compensation, but that greater success can be achieved when one is young. The reason is there are fewer psychological stress patterns to resist, which even block treatment.

Not for nought it is said that, "you are your doctor's bank account"; for if they keep you ill they are in business for life – *their* life. Their materialistic attitude only makes it is harder for them to be objective. Objectivity would require them to open themselves to new recognitions and to share common and logical findings.

One would expect that those sure of their convictions would let fact speak against fact. Oh no! Doctors intentionally avoid such discourses because they feel and know that what they have studied and hold so dear are but the cognitive claims of others they have so far obeyed. So medical professionals choose to continue closing themselves to any ideas not borne within their circles. But such arrogance and conceit come from fear. A fear of it becoming known that what they have accepted as truth and upheld as gospel is but a platform ready to be ripped away from under them.

Fear can also cause one, cognisant of another with a higher recognition, to become filled with hatred. An open declaration of one's inferior mind, giving rise to the propensity of envy toward the other that can comprehend something which to him or her remains incomprehensible.

The more influence such individuals exert upon society, and the more they realise that the public may learn of this deficient knowledge, the more energetically will they close themselves to recognition, especially from an outside source. And the more desperately will they work against this source in order to save face, from fear of being treated with disdain in public opinion, thus lose power and affluence.

With arrogance and vanity, these intellectuals unfoundedly challenge other perspectives often-times with hatred and tyranny.

They are quick to ostracise others capable of higher recognitions from their circles. They question the credentials of those who do not belong among their intellectual circles and label them "charlatans" and "quacks", stopping at nothing to eliminate them, to force them to live under constant threat of jail for practicing medicine without a license.

With the power given to them by the State, medical professionals feel they have the right to enforce upon us their chosen practice of medicine, after all, they spent at least seven years in medical school, although with only a few curriculum hours given to nutrition. While they play "god" with our health, the masses look on, "neutered", void of the knowledge to form a conviction to demand the right path to holistic well-being. They offer no support to those who risk their freedom to preserve the methods of Natural Medicine which developed through our close relations with Nature. One need not look far to see the sad havoc such wrong attitude has brought about - one new disease after the other, societies with staggering public health care bills.

PART TWO

THE TEMPERAMENT

As discussed in Part I, the union of the radiations of ethereal matter with fine dense matter gives rise to the different species of human temperament – the specific patterns of response of the nervous system to internal and external stimuli; partly genetically inherited and the other, of the nature of one's urges of the soul. The temperament is basically how the nervous system reacts, characterising one's particular individuality. What, therefore, does the temperament have to do with organic conditions when it is already established that symbionts, *etc.*, are what cause pathological diseases?

First let us look at the definition of temperament: "the characteristic phenomena of an individual's emotional nature, including his susceptibility to emotional stimulation, his customary strength and speed of response, the quality of his prevailing mood, and all peculiarities of fluctuation and intensity in mood; these phenonmena being regarded as dependent upon constitutional makeup, and therefore largely hereditary in origin."[16]

Essentially, temperament expresses the relationship of humans to the events going on around them. It is important, however, to distinguish temperament, character and personality, in order to avoid confusion.

According to the *Great Soviet Encyclopedia, 3rd* Edition: Character is defined as the "valuable and constant individual mould of spiritual life of man, its type, and all the 'ethics' of man, which show themselves in individual acts and states of his psychological life, as well as his manners, habits, frame of mind and the circle of emotional life peculiar to him. The character of man forms the basis of his behavior ..."

Our temperament and character analyses reveal our personality. The same text defined personality as: "the integrating starting-point, which combines the different psychological processes of the individual into a stage unit and which gives behavior an inevitable sequence and stability." But Pavlov, the Russian scientist sums up the three variables quite beautifully when he wrote: "The personality of man is determined by biological inheritance as well as environment. The strength of the nervous system (temperament) is an innate property, while character (form of behavior) is mainly comprised of acquired habits."[17]

This study of body-mind relation finds its historical roots as far back as ancient Egypt. Later, ancient Greek physicians formulated the mind-body relation from the point of view of the influence of bodily conditions upon behavior. Two concepts were of primary importance: the *humors* (body fluids) and *pneuma* (vital spirit).

The humoral theory gave rise to the concept of the temperament, which Hippocrates (500 B.C), the father of medicine, and others have deemed part of a medical theory of life. These distinguished physicians positioned the pneuma (related to the basic element or principle, air (breath), and to life itself) to explain many physiological processes, including mental activity.

In one of his treatises, Hippocrates wrote: "the pneuma or vital spirit is supposed to circulate through the blood vessels and carry sensation itself." Hence his development of the term temperament - the balance in an individual between the various humors.

He determined that the psychological disposition of man, the individual features of his behavior, could be determined by the relationship of four humors (fluid media) with the body: blood, phlegm, black bile, and yellow bile. These fluids designated specific temperament – the one most predominant creates an imbalance in the body whereby the individual brings the predisposition to certain organic diseases. After a time, however, by the second century A.D., the doctrine of these ascribed humors proved misleading and was later attributed to wet, dry, warm and cold physical conditions, and practised as part of medicine well into the nineteenth century. Until, of course, the materialist and his extolled doctrine, that Dense Matter (the body) is primary of all that exists and spirit is a product, entered the high edifice of medicine.

The four basic temperament are also attributed to the names of four Greek gods, said to be responsible for forming humans: Dionysus (gives the gift of a free spirit, joy); Epimenthean (gives a sense of duty, social conscience); Promethean (gives the gift of science); and Apollonian (gives the spiritual quest for things beyond material existence/self-actualisation). In another branch of learning, the empirical classifications which still exist up to today, placed the temperament groups in which humanity is divided – *the sanguine, the melancholic, the choleric* and *the phlegmatic* types which also correspond to the four human life cycles: the sanguine, which resembles childhood, the freedom loving, impetuous individual; the melancholic, which resembles youth – endowed with a sense duty – poised always to take action; the choleric, which resembles matured manhood and womanhood cycle of fiery action; and the phlegmatic, the reflective type, resembling the final life-cycle which synthesises one's mature deed for posterity.

And what Galen (131 - 201 A.D.) claimed explicitly about the influence of the humors on individual personality differences remains gospel whether one accepts it or not. He said: "Those who do not consider that the mind is helped or harmed by the bodily crasis [constitutional temperament] can tell nothing about the differences in children, nor can they explain the help we derive from diet; nor again why there are so many differences in character, some individuals appearing spirited, others spiritless, some intelligent and others not so."

The Temperament and the Blood

The temperament works through the blood, in other words, it radiates the blood. The spirit forms the human blood, in accordance with the kind of activities in which we choose to engage ourselves. Spirit cannot express itself in the field of action (matter) except directly through the blood, the great difference between the two species (spirit and matter) and prevents this, it can only become outwardly active through the radiation of the blood.

The temperament therefore, forms the actual bridge for the performance of our highest achievements, but then, only if the blood is of a very particular composition suitable for the soul concerned. In accordance with the blood-composition there will always be a type of temperament most distinct which is decisive for each individual. The four different blood compositions, groups O, A, B and AB, which speak to the evolutionary self-conscious development of the different human species, are the basic groups the entire human race classifies itself, indicating different spiritual maturity as expressed in the four basic temperament.

Therefore, the accustomed division of societies and races into class structure instead of the homogenous blood types – as it has to do with the shared gifts and abilities – points to one of the fundamental reasons behind the ongoing disputatious and disharmony whether in intimate relationships, family, workplace or society-at-large based on incompatible mixing of blood-types. Still, the different blood DNA profiles point also to the fact that even within this homogeneity, there are hardly any two people alike in blood formula – individuality, which again points back to the fact it is our spiritual nature which has the ruling influence behind all our perceptions, thoughts and actions.

There are other factors, however, which further influence the characteristics of the different peoples: their regions of origin and everything pertaining to them, *i.e.*, climate, the radiation of the stars, the different kinds of nourishment, but most of all, the maturity of the particular soul itself. Still we are not purely of one definite temperament, but bear certain elements of the basic four types. But with all the admixtures, there is a consequent ideal temperament that is predominant. The more spiritually matured is the individual the more readily discernable in personality is this primary temperament.

From this primary temperament in one's personality, an observer can anticipate rather accurately what one will do most of the time. The temperament is that which places a signature on each of our actions, making it recognisably our own. But as the physical body ages the blood-composition also changes. With healthy blood, an increasing age comes with a corresponding change of the temperament. When the composition changes, this naturally alters the radiation, producing therewith corresponding alternating effects upon the person concerned as well as upon our environment.

Hence the change of the blood-composition from childhood to adolescent cycle, which is not just to be observed by the visible change of form of the physical body, but the mental peculiarities of an individual as manifest in one's reaction to particular stimuli or influences within the environment, in other words, one's behavioral pattern.

Sickness, however, prevents this logical development, for it brings confusion to the radiations. The same person who, in one state of health is irritable, violent, passional, even sensual and cruel, who in good physical and psychic condition, is amiable, even-tempered, moral and good.

The Blood Circulation

Adolescence therefore, is that time when the spirit begins to contribute to the changing of the blood-composition from that of childhood; the process marks the gradual awakening of generative power. The secret of this transformation lies in the blood as formed by the human spirit, allowing the talents and abilities to proceed and develop in the proper manner. As young adults we are then able to master our talent, absorb it completely until it becomes second nature. Hence the saying: "it becomes flesh and blood". What this means is that it not only becomes comprehension with the "fleshy" brain, but also a grasping with the spirit, which can only come into the field of action by expressing through the blood-radiation.

Of what significance therefore is the human blood if it plays so major apart in character development? Use an incubating egg as an example. Experiment shows that the larger part is warmer than the other parts, because its vitality is there, which if cold life is extinct; incubate it for a short time, and break the shell at the larger end and we will see the heart palpating and blood-vessels, the yoke furnishing the required nutrition. The vital apparatus forms first, and deposits the material for forming to the other portions.

What is worth noting, however, is that the incubation process is most active during the juvenility stage of development. What develops in this cycle along with the tiny blood vessels sustains the whole animal economy; is the source of all power and energy that creates animal heat; resists cold and heat, disease and death; and re-supplies muscles, brain, and nerve that life power expended by the very exertion. Hence generative power is to adolescence what fire, fuel, water, and steam are to machinery - "the *vis animae the primum mobile* - the first prerequisite of life itself and all its functions" (Fowler).

Whereas the philosopher Emanuel Kant attached great importance to the individual features of the blood, it is not difficult to understand why others, like Russian physiologist P. F. Lesgaft, placed importance on the blood vessels. The forming of the blood vessels marks the source of power to begin life, more importantly, spiritual life. The aorta (main artery) divided into a number of main branches, is in turn divided into smaller ones until the entire body is supplied by an elaborately branching series of blood vessels. The smallest arteries divide into a fine network of still more minute vessels, called capillaries, which through their extremely thin walls enable the blood to come into close relation with the fluids and tissues of the body.

In the capillaries, the blood performs three functions: releases its oxygen to the tissues; furnishes to the body cells the nutrients and other essential substances that it carries; and takes up waste products from the tissues. The capillaries then unite to form small veins, which in turn unite to form larger veins until the blood is finally collected into the superior and inferior venae cavae which take it to the heart, completing the circuit. But if the blood vessels are damaged one can only see how life-force is restricted and can eventually lead to death.

And so it is, that even though the embryo bears life in form, not until that definite stage of pregnancy – mid-way through – does the unborn child begin to form a personality. The incarnation of the spirit, which is signalled by the child's first movement, called a "kick", is the actual moment its own blood begins to circulate; whereas at physical death, when the spirit has left the body, the blood ceases to pulsate and exist altogether, only it's congealed residue remains in the veins.

Hence, the blood is only present during the time between the entrance and departure of the spirit, when the spirit dwells inside the body. In traumatic incidences causing a lack of blood the spirit must therefore finally sever its connection with its physical body, *i.e.*, death occurs. The person is said, "to bleed to death."

While the blood is the life of the soul itself, it is also the great porter of the system; it carries away all the material with which to build up and repair every part, and hurries off the waste material, which it expels through the lungs and skin. Hence, without the heart, even the lungs could not function, or vice-versa. They are the co-workers at the fountain-head of life. Even the diseased organs are unloaded of morbid matter, reanimated, and rebuilt mainly by the blood. Therefore blood good or poor, the entire system, the brain included, is in a good or poor condition; blood wanting, all is wanting; heart poor, all is poor; heart improved, all is improved.

It is for this reason the sanguine temperament which forms primal life is associated with the blood and corresponds to the O Blood type – the most primitive blood group. All the other blood groups carry the O antigen. Active blood, bloodthirsty, full-blooded and meanings attributed to sanguine. The child develops best when it is sanguine, therefore the blood is such as to produce the sanguine temperament. This allows for the undimmed joy of the moment; warmth in the character; impulsiveness; the liability to overdo and passional excesses. So regardless of one's blood type, we all bear the "O" type child within, which at times needs to be free; freedom to act without fetter or constraint. To enjoy every moment, for tomorrow with its cares and responsibilities never comes.

Then comes early manhood and womanhood (adolescence), in which the melancholic temperament, connected to kidney function, which concerns our feelings and desires. Symbolically the kidney "expresses externally that which is within". The melancholic cycle is the best time for maturing. If grounded in the right upbringing it can direct the spirit towards purity and loyalty, at which time it takes an active lead and gears into the development and the expression of gifts and abilities. Hence the healthy daydreams in which adolescents indulge and their passion to improve the world, ambitions which are usually muffled by adults who themselves have had an arrested adolescent development.

Thereafter comes the years of man's and woman's full estate which is the choleric temperament, connected to the liver, the organ of equanimity and sanity. It marks the stage of human development when the spirit should be in its clarified form, which is needed for the full execution of action. At this time the spirit *must* dominate, it must ennoble and transfigure everything, it must send out powerful thoughts, words and actions in Creation.

And finally comes old-age, the phlegmatic temperament, connected to the movement of phlegm, the lymphatic system. Hence the cycle when the immune system is put to its test, with diseases of old-age, mostly auto immune diseases. This is the cycle for quiet reflection, the time when material things should no longer be of importance. We re-examine past experiences of life in order to retain the lessons learned. If one has lived a fulfilled life there is no longer the fear of death, little by little the soul detaches itself from the body.

And all of these cycles must be experienced at the required time. Each must close at the beginning of the other, spiritually, mentally and physically, whereby at old-age there comes a smooth releasing or a severance of earth-life, called death.

The period of early manhood and womanhood or puberty is classified as the age of the melancholic temperament, because only as the spirit breaks through in the generative powers does it find a direct connection with the species of Creation. Here the young adult ego begins to mediate between the *sanguine* and the *choleric,* of which neither extremes can be removed. Though chided by childish indulgences, the youths feel compelled to more meaningful actions. They become responsible for their deeds in Creation, fully responsible for every thought, for every word, and for every action, because all the vibrations thereof are pressing in full power, thereby penetrating the animistic, *i.e.*, elemental faculties and producing form – the yolk furnishing the required nutrition –the prerequisite for life itself and all its functions. Responsibility, the inherent nature of spirit, is what separates human behavior from that of the child or animal.

The organic condition of the blood, therefore, is what lies behind and below all the human temperament — are, indeed, their determining cause. And organic hereditary quality is that which is called "bottom" in horse, "the breed" in full-blooded animals, and "blood" in those high and nobly born. Hence the saying "It runs in the blood". For it is the organic blood conditions of the attracting parents' blood which determine the form of the physical body and its accompanying manner of movement, as well as the mental proclivities and their controlling influence on character. All humans conform to the particular species, that is, the genetic quality to which one is attracted or deserves, the Law to which everyone is subject.

The doctrine of the temperament underwent many changes and showed up in behavioral psychology as character types in the science of phrenology – derived from the Greek words relating to mind and discourse. The phrenological theory of brain structure was originated by German physician Franz Joseph Gall (1758-1823). Its later philosophy declares that, with a growth in the faculties through exercise, a person can consciously develop and cultivate his virtues, *i.e.*, socially desirable propensities, and restrain his vices, *i.e.*, overdeveloped, socially undesirable propensities. In explaining how the human mind in directly affected by bodily health, it points out certain cause and effect relations existing between particular forms or development of the brain, and their accompanying manifestations of mind, and predicates the respective peculiarities of the character and talents of different persons from the forms, sizes, and other organic conditions of their brains.

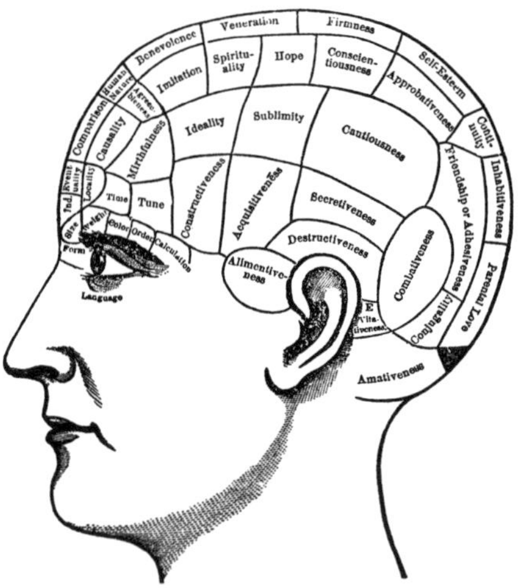

Thirty-seven faculties: the phrenological "organs"

For the purpose of classification the human race was divided into four basic psychological types: the "nervous" or melancholic, distinguished by large brain, delicate health, and emaciation; the "bilious" or choleric, harsh features and firm muscles; the "sanguine", large lung capacity and moderate plumpness; and the "lymphatic", rounded form and heavy countenance.

Phrenologists refined the four original types to three essential components making up the structure of temperament: the general activity of the individual, his motive forces, and emotionality, hence a body form bearing a definite disposition where there is a predominance. Thus we have the classification and definition of the three basic body-types – the *vital,* the *motive,* the *mental*; the sanguine and choleric temperament considered variants of the motive; melancholic, the mental; and phlegmatic, the vital. The doctrine concurs:

> Man is composed of three great classes of organs, the predominance or deficiency of each of which is called a predominant or deficient temperament, each giving a particular form to the body – shape being its index, – and likewise a particular set of phrenological developments, and consequent traits of character. This is, given forms of body indicate and accompany special talents, dispositions, and mental proclivities; and the art of delineating phrenological character depends in a great degree on reading correctly the temperament and organic conditions, and their controlling influence on character; for they exert, as it were, the ground-swell as to the direction and action of the phrenological manifestations. Thus Causality, with the vital temperament predominant takes on the phase of planning, of common sense, of reasoning on matter, of adapting ways and means to ends, but with the nervous or mental predominant, the same Causality manifests itself in logic, metaphysics, in investigation, the origination of ideas, in intellectual clearness and power, and it requires the sharpest eye and clearest head in the examiner to discern the bearings and influences of these temperamental and organic conditions on the intellectual and moral manifestations. And the mistakes of the amateurs, of connoisseurs even, are more temperamental than phrenological. Still they are sometimes consequent on health conditions. Thus the same person in one state of health is irritable, violent, passional, perhaps even sensual and wicked, who in another physical condition is amiable, even-tempered, moral, and good. A given amount of ideality is

much more ideal, of language much more expressive, of the affections more affectional, and moral tone more lofty, in combination with the mental temperament than vital. But our proposed limits do not allow us to extend our observations. Still, the following descriptions give the outline, and put inquirers on the track of further observations.

The classification of the three bodily temperament (forms) accordingly to phrenology – the vital, motive and mental – remains, however, subordinate to the study of the nature of personality – the sanguine, melancholic, choleric and phlegmatic. Bodily classifications are but the mechanical actions and work of the physical body, whereas the personality actually "leads" in these things, to that which is willed by the spirit and which the brain and the bodily implements then turn into action. Hence, the higher nervous (psychological) behavior should be noticed first, and when the bodily texture or form is either coarse, strong, fine or soft the brain will correspond with that of the body, and mental characteristics with that of the brain. Classifications, however, are for the purpose of exposition and are not mutually exclusive, a mix in varying proportions more the rule.

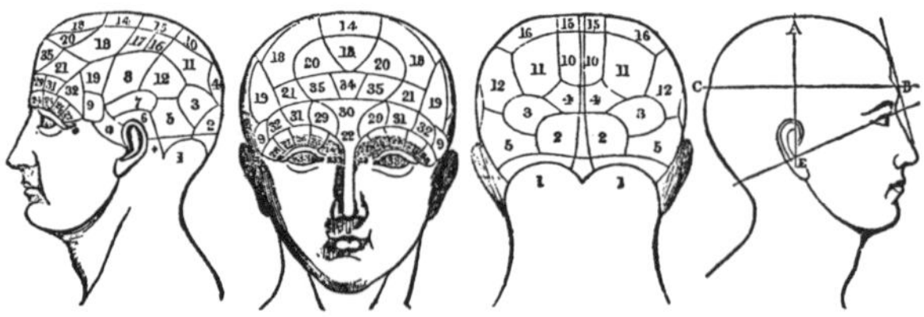

Numbered divisions of the brain

This bodily temperament embraces the heart, lungs, stomach, liver, bowels, and that entire system of internal organs which creates life-force.

ALIMENTATION: The Absorption and Assimilation of Nutrients

Optimum function of the vital organs and systems depends upon Alimentation. Since we are all born with different body chemistries and the way we have treated our bodies determines different rates of digestion and assimilation, should there not be a comprehensive, physiological analysis of each individual's body chemistry to determine one's ability to digest and assimilate nutrients? The facts can only answer affirmatively.

If it is otherwise, we will not be successful in getting to the root of symptoms and be able to detect alterations and correct them with the correct choice of foods, and whole food complexes such as plant enzymes. If these alterations are not corrected, the body will try to compensate endogenously, that is, "rob Peter to pay Paul". When this ability to compensate is exhausted, it must alter the body's function to sustain itself; it produces symptoms, without physical findings. If this process continues uncorrected, the altered body's function changes tissue structure. Disharmony sets in – joint damage, tumors, *etc.* – all mostly irreversible.

Manager's Syndrome

The hyperexcitability caused by stress in the modern world has only led to disorder of the autonomic nerve function. The result is nervous diseases results from toxic irritation of the neurones. *Dyspepsia*, which is common among business people, is more a mental or nervous than physical disease, although this is presumed to be the other way around, in that, most stomach ulcer patients carry a common bacteria known as *Helicobacter pylori*, which is "presumably" killed with antibiotics. One of the condition which causes the development of bacteria and other stomachtic is a worried, feverish, unhappy state of mind, which cannot be corrected permanently with antacids or anitbiotics.

Most of the time dyspepsia is brought on by eating hurriedly and too much, which allows so little energy to go the stomach, that its contents ferment instead of being digested, which inflames the whole system, and causes morbid action in both the mental and physical functions. This inflammation co-creates a craving, hankering appetite, as well as a generally irritable state of mind. And the more food is eaten the more it re-inflames the stomach, increasing these morbid hankerings; while one finds denying the appetite diminishes this inflammation and consequent hungering and irritability. Sometimes eating gives temporary relief right before what has just been eaten ferments, but only increases the pain soon afterwards.

Starvation is the cure in all cases of craving appetite. This situation can be easily remedied if we avoid eating in a hurried, anxious state. We should eat as if determined to enjoy it; above all, casting off care, dispel grief, business anxieties, troubles, and all painful memories and anticipations, and just luxuriate in the moment.

A comparison of humans and animals shows that the latter does not overfeed its body as humans do. It is satisfied when it no longer feels hungry, whereas in many cases humans are not satisfied until they can eat no more. The animals also drink only to quench thirst. Humans, however, live under the illusion that to enjoy oneself, this must be carried to the excess - consuming more alcohol, stimulants such as coffee and tea to the excess - forsaking water - Nature's most luxurious drink.

It is recommended to make it a habit to rub and pat, or lightly pound the stomach, liver, and bowels. This supplies that mechanical action which restores them to normal function. Those manual exercises, such as rowing, chopping wood, hoeing, especially the yogic abdominal lifts, which call the abdominal muscles into special attention, are preeminently useful.

But there must be a compulsion to achieve this well-being. As soon as there arises the sincere and ardent desire to change the wrong manner of eating, the spirit will govern the process and bring about the fulfilment of this intention. We arrive at the point where our sensitivity is heightened to all the happenings within the body. We become aware of the effects particular foods have on body and spirit, by noting the way we feel. This state of maturity is the only guide against the compulsive habit of overeating. And in this parents and guardians will guide children in the right manner.

THE VITAL CIRCULATORY SYSTEM

The human organism has three circulatory systems – the cardiovascular, the lymphatic, and the nervous impulses. For the vital temperament, the cardiovascular system, which is just as important as the lymphatic and nervous systems are closely linked, as in a triad.

The heart pumps up to 5,000 gallons of blood a day, under pressure, through the network of arteries, veins and capillaries. the heart is formed during the fetal stage by tapping the energies of the soul. Hence its close connection to the ethereal body, from which pure love vibration emanates. Failure to express the love energies at the higher level, automatically give rise to a symbolic appropriate problem at the physical level, such as congenital damage. When the heart problem is in the form of heart attack, usually due to failure of the blood supply to the heart muscle, it is said that the symbolic indicator is that such an individual has not supplied the love side of his "triangle" with sufficient energy, in that blood equals energy.

CHRONIC CONSTIPATION AND THE HEART

Constipation is considered the most chronic gastrointestinal complaint. Apart from too much undigested toxic-waste protein lying in the lower bowels, the condition may exist on a deeper level. It may have to do with the extracellular (cell exterior) fluid, due to weakness of the heart. This fluid is composed of:

1. 75% Interstital Fluid (within the tissues), containing very little protein.
2. 25% Blood Plasma, which uses protein for osmotic pressure in maintaining the plasma volume, and contains 7.5% of total body water. If plasma water is reduced for whatever reason, plasma protein will compete with intracellular (cell interior) protein for

water and gradually draw water out of the cells. This is one of the ways circulatory volume is maintained and thirst is stimulated.

Distribution between the extracellular fluids and the blood plasma is maintained by plasma protein which draws water into circulation. It is balanced by the hydorstatic pressure of the heart which drives water out of the plasma. A loss of plasma protein allows more plasma water to escape into the extracellular space.

However, a weak heart may create a backward failure (hold water in the plasma) and increase the hydrostatic pressure in the veins, pulling water into the extracellular spaces causing the condition called, hypertonic ECF. This gives rise constipation and liver dysfunction – portal vein congestion (varicose veins), dyskinesia of the bile duct, hemorrhoids.

The plasma then becomes hypertonic, urine volume increases. To compensate, the pituitary osmoreceptors are continuously stimulated to release the antidiuretic hormone (ADH) or vasopressin from the adrenals to reabsorb the water, to dilute the blood and concentrate the urine. This should lower ECF tonicity. But a weak heart causes an overstimulation of vasopressin and eventually exhaust the adrenal. For as water leaves the cells, the disturbance of the osmotic pressure gradient causes electrolytes (chloride, sodium, and potassium) to enter the cells. The adrenals then has to secrete aldosterone, a diuretic hormone which balances the salt-water ratio in the body, which it cannot do adequately if exhausted. Symptoms of adrenal cortisol (aldosterone) insufficiency are: weakness, anorexia, weight loss, nausea, vomiting, hypotension,. symptoms of hypoglycemia, pigmentation.

This can lead to kidney failure due to insufficient loss of electrolytes. If excess potassium is retained by the body, it causes blood alkalinity. Symptoms include: anxiety, agitation, severe weakness, fatigue; hyporeflexia (poor reflexes), paralysis of extremities, effect on heart; early signs includes: peaked T waves, later, widening of QRS and P-R interval). Most cases of hyperkalemia (high concentration of potassium in the blood) are due to renal failure,

Spironolactone (synthetic corticosteriod hormone) diuretic or Addison disease.

So a weak heart may indicate to kidney failure, which leads to dyskinesia (backup) of the liver and bile ducts, which leads to pancreas irritation. This creates what is medically called, the liver-heart-kidney syndrome.

For this reason bowel conditions are related to issues of the heart, on the astral (emotional) level as well as on the physical. As previously stated, impressions entering the solar plexus radiate upon the heart. The governing endocrine gland of the solar plexus is the pancreas – and its other mesenteries in the digestive process: the stomach, gall-bladder, liver and the small intestines – and their dysfunction radiate back upon the heart and vice-versa.

When the spiritual radiations of the solar plexus are balanced, the experience is determination, assertion, personal power, hearty laughter; when unbalanced, the experience is lack of will power, brute propensity, anger, fear, hate. These experiences radiate upon its higher counterpart – the heart energy centre (chakra), which concerns unconditional love, forgiveness, people consciousness, peace, tolerance,

When we suppress the true feelings of the heart whether from our negative attitude or not effectively deal with karmic issues in our lives and how we learn from them, the result is a blockage or suppression of energies – a spiritual drought which prevents us from expressing our talents to the best of our abilities. We cannot help becoming trapped in our survival-consciousness mode. This is the root of our anger, resentment, self-pity – to the point of lovelessness, and related heart problems. And these negative energies flow back to the solar plexus-digestive centre, which in turn inhibits the flow of digestive secretions and normal nerve impulses to the bowels, causing constipation (the drought effect). It could also be heart-digestive problems relating to such conditions as meteorism (bloating) and congestive gastritis, resulting in poor digestion and related eating disorders.

The inflammation caused by dyspepsia, ulcer, or undigested food sitting in the stomach is enough to cause morbid action in both mental and physical function. Apart from anger and irritability, this inflamed state is what creates a craving, hankering appetite. And the more food is eaten the more it re-inflames the stomach. The creative love energy is then brought down from its lofty heights to the sensual indulgence, in this case to appease the senses with more food, usually the wrong choice – carbohydrates, more the refined ("junk-food") than the wholesome complex group.

PROTECTING YOUR HEART

- If you smoke, stop. Nicotine raises the pulse and blood pressure and, with carbon dioxide, adds to the risk of clotting.
- Change your diet; avoid fatty foods, sugar, excess salt, which all link to arterial disease.
- Exercise regularly, this improves your heart performance.
- Maintain normal body weight to prevent strain on the heart.
- Practice relaxation and therapies such as meditation, yoga, nature walks, to combat stress.
- Learn to exercise patience and forbearance.
- Banish worry, doubt and fear.
- Above all, express always the Christ-love; that which harbors no resentment or hatred.

The Law Of Breath

All that lives, even vegetables and trees, breathes, must breathe in order to live, and live in proportion as they breathe; begin life's first function with breathing and end its last with the last breath. Whereas blood remains the most important element of life, breathing is the most important function – from the first breath to the last – it is the grand stimulator and sustainer of all. Therefore, without the heart, the lungs would be irrelevant, and vice-versa.

It is of this co-creative act Hippocrates made reference, that pneuma, the breath of life or vital spirit is supposed to circulate through the blood vessels and carry sensation itself. Modern medical research has uncovered that it is the sinus nerves which help to retain this consciousness and power to "experience". Hence more and more the relation of respiration to behavior and its disorders in being recognised in the scientific world. Various investigations have been carried out and enough data gathered regarding modifications of breathing in attention, mental effort and in various emotional and other patterns of behavior.

Therefore, gaining knowledge of the law of breath is of critical importance, not only to regulate behavior, but also, according to many authorities on the breathing practice, help attain purification of mind and body. In fact, many feel that no other practice is necessary. For this reason correct breathing forms part of the matrix in body alignment, for the eradication of all toxins from the body.

The alvoelar surface (the air sacs at the end of each bronchiole) in the lungs is by far the most excitable within the visceral cavity (including the stomach, lungs, heart, *etc.*) and together with the bronchi, trachea, larynx and the nose, form the best medium to attain a fluid movement or involuntary activity of the intuitively dominated sympathetic nerve branch essential for maintaining a homeostatic balance. The involuntary reactions working through the respiratory mechanism maintain the fluidity of the cerebellum. Hence the stimulation of the respiratory systems involves a distinct, higher level of nervous (psychological) activity.

The controlling areas of respiration lay beyond the phrenic nerve – the primary motor nerves of the cervical plexus – the principal respiratory nerve of the body leading to the diaphragm (the chief muscle of respiration), involving the involuntary (automatic) and voluntary (cerebrospinal) impulses through the control of respiration; higher than the controlling area of the pons and the medulla; higher than the hypothalamic level which controls the autonomic nervous system. It reaches up to the medial, basal and sub-cortical areas of the midbrain – the topmost structure of the brain stem which contains major relay stations for neurons transmitting signals to the cerebral cortex, as well as many reflex centres – pathways carrying sensory or astral (input) information and motor (output) commands.

And to this effect medical research has uncovered that the sinus nerves help to retain this consciousness and power to "experience". According to yogic literature, the internal carotid helps retention of consciousness by feeding the brain with the requisite amount of blood and are therefore our consciousness producers. It is for this function the brain requires a high amount of oxygen and glucose, which are supplied by way of the carotids.

One can now understand the adverse effect toxins in blood (which are deposited in the brain) has upon human conscious awareness. When compressed hard and long by toxic overload, these internal carotids become "stupor producers", *i.e.,* producers of gross stupidity or indolence.

The carotid sinuses also regulate blood pressure and heart rate, hence the liver-kidney-heart syndrome from their compression. More and more, the relation of respiration to behavior and its disorders is being recognised in the scientific world. Various investigations have been carried out and enough data gathered regarding the effect modification of breathing has on attention, mental effort and various emotional and other patterns of behavior.

Studies have linked somatic conditions like pulmonary tuberculosis and asthma with personality conflicts and such conflicts are now presumed important factors in the onset and course of these diseases.[18] Just compare the jerky and rapid breathing and movement of mice, which have one of the shortest life spans, to the methodical movement of the tortoise with one of the longest life-spans and you will see this correlation of breath to radiant health. Harriet, the Australian tortoise was still alive in December, 1997, at the golden age of 167. Of course, the two examples are the extreme, in that, one displays exaggerated movement and the other, is characterised by movement which is too slow. However, this analogy was used for the purpose of observing the anxious lives of many, and apart from their states of ill-health, the mistakes and failures their works produce, compared to those who are at peace with themselves and whose work bears lasting effects from having found the simplicity of a happy medium - and that the law of breath is a principle which must be consciously applied.

CONTROLLED AND PROLONGED RESPIRATION

The breathing art, however, speaks to volitional controlled breathing, not merely that of forced deep inspirations and expirations. Controlled and prolonged respiration as that of yogic breathing. A discipline practice that can be cultivated: by first breathing deeply and rapidly (snapping breath); then draw long and full breaths; filling the lungs at every inspiration. At such times we should dress loosely and, preferably, sit erect (cross legged if possible), so that the diaphragm can allow extra lung action; begin and maintain an extra exertion with extra lung action; see how many deep full breaths you can comfortably take; ventilate your rooms, especially sleeping quarters, well, and be much of the time in open air. Everywhere try to cultivate full and frequent lung inflation, by breathing clear out, clear in, and low down; that is, make all your breathing as when taking a long breath.

According to Fowler, breathing as fast and as much fresh air as possible, and in few hours can "reverse and prevent" the worst attack of disease you can have; for this will both unload disease at every pore of skin and lungs, and infuse into the system that *vis animae* which will both grapple with and expel the disease in all its forms, and restore health, strength and life. Nature has no panacea like breath.

Even in the cases of the blues, he cited deep breathing can easily and quickly dispel them, especially if we add vigorous exercise. In keeping our lungs clear up to their fullest, liveliest action, we deepen and quicken our divine inspiration and put forth our greatest mental exertions in speaking or writing. We can only breathe forth your highest, holiest orisions of thanksgiving and worship by deepening our inspiration of fresh air and, fully enjoy bodily pleasures in copious breathing. In short, deep, copious breathing is the alpha and omega of all physical, and thereby of all mental and moral function and enjoyment.

Based on the research of the late Dr. Vinekar (1907-1967) of India, yogic type breathing claims volitional breathing not merely to clean the sinus nerves ...

> But can effect a change in the very pathways and impulses through the brain, resulting in a constant steadiness and balance of mind... By Parayamas (controlled breath), that are practised correctly, the whole nervous system is well integrated and then the impulses run easily through the 'susumma' - the central tract - after clearing away the occlusion that had erstwhile blocked this pathway. The impulses coursing thus through the central pathway give rise to a steadiness (and balance) of mind. (H.Y.P. II 41-42).
>
> The circuit of these impulses, they say, normally runs through the 'lateral regions', and this course of it gives rise to ego-centricism and unsteadiness of mind. If instead, the impulses were to course the 'central circuit', that would contribute to peace and mental balance. Then, the mental energies could be controlled easily and canalized for higher ends. Normally, however, this central path remains blocked by 'kapha'[19] , but Pranayama, especially in Bhastrika variety, helps to break these 'obstructions' and render the passage free, *i.e.*, it helps to activate the same ... H.Y.P II-65-66).

Here we can see the relation of breath to the condition of fibrosis: pulmonary interstitial – the thickening and stiffening of the lining of the air sacs (alveoli) of the lungs; cystic – tissue growth and inflammation of the endocrine glands; endometriosis – tissue growth affecting the lining of the uterus and surrounding sites, causing continuous pain, and the growth of fibroids and cysts, *etc.*, - pointing to the relation of the female endocrine system and a woman's mental and nervous states which, hereditary or not, leads back to the functioning of the digestive system. And not one of these conditions of the digestive system and smooth muscles can be corrected without paying attention to "pneuma" – the breath of life.

Dr. Vinekar continues:

> It will be of interest here to note that, recently, Dr. Heath of the Tulane University, and his colleagues working on the problems of schizophrenia, have postulated a similar hypothesis of two separate circuits in the brain: (1) a facilitatory circuit coursing through the septal region, and (2) an inhibitory one, working through the lateral regions [0] The hypothesis is being tested on human beings, who could 'talk out of their minds', with electrode implantation in sub-cordial regions for over a year and stimulation of these regions through deep leads. This latter technique, however, is still crude, according to them and not very satisfactory. Yet, the work done so far has been enough to indicate a possibility of the two circuits postulated by them.
>
> The 'Central Circuit' implied by our ancient Yogins may not exactly be the septal one. (They claim that along with the activation of the 'central circuit', there is also a cessation of breathing).
>
> To be more exact, the ancient adepts in Yoga postulated two latent brain circuits in human beings, (1) Central Circuit - 'madhya patha' - (2) Superior Circuit - 'urdhapatha'. 'Samadhi[20] stage is supposed to set in when the latter is activated. It is very difficult to locate these on mere neuro-anatomical grounds.
>
> Yet, if we take into consideration the supramedullary pathways of respiratory innervation, the empirical claim of these adepts that Pranayama can activate new circuits of impulses seems to be quite plausible. It has, however, to be put to a very severe test and investigation, and the method of a multi-disciplinary approach, that is followed by the Tulane University group of scientists, if applied to the

investigation on some advanced students of Yoga, should perhaps be expected to go a long way to test and explain in a rational way the claim made by the ancient Yogic adepts.

Patanjali claims that judicious Pranayama can break the barriers that are responsible to keep us in the darkness, *i.e.*, it can open up the doors that would lead us to self-realisation ...

CONTROLLED BREATH

Exercise:

This volitional, controlled breathing is not merely that of breathing exercises forcing deep inspirations and expirations, but controlled and prolonged respiration as in yogic breathing. This practice can be cultivated by first breathing deeply and rapidly for a few seconds (increase time gradually) what is called snapping breath; then draw long and full breaths; fill your lungs at every inspiration, effortlessly retain, breath - definite proportion of time governed by your capacity so as not to transgress your own limitations and wreck the delicate and vital mechanism of respiration and through it the whole organismic function; empty lungs completely at every expiration; not only heave the chest in breathing, but also work the abdomen.

There is no set rule of timing proportions for the inspiration, retention and expiration, but if one so chooses, a common ratio is 1 : 4 : 2 mental counts – giving yourself as much time as possible to retain and double the time to expiration as to inspiration. This ratio, however, could prove quite drastic as a beginner, hence one may gradually develop a unique pattern – a ratio count like a 1 : 1 : 2, through a slow and gradual development to say, 1 : 4 : 2, or whatever feels most comfortable.

The main thing to keep in mind is that the deep breathing process must be effortless. This point cannot be over-stressed; there should be no "hunger" for air at any stage of controlled breathing. The respiratory mechanism remains a delicate balance in the medulla; any tampering with this balance can only lead to tragic results, physically and psychologically.

Refined Carbohydrates – Their Effects on Vital Temperament

Refined carbohydrates by their very nature sap generative power. Such is the consumption of heavy, rich, processed, fried, refined and devitalized foods, which only overwork the digestive system, liver and pancreas, channeling the generative power along with the blood away from all other parts of the body, rendering the individual physically, mentally and spiritually inept. Such is a violation of the Law of Continuous Movement.

An overindulgence in refined carbohydrates (starch) such as sugar, flour, and white rice depletes essential nutrients, especially vitamins. A deficiency in B vitamins not only impairs the conversion of carbohydrates into energy, but protein and fat metabolism as well.

A deficiency of B vitamins causes poor protein metabolism. A percentage of the body's protein is converted to glucose, which is the only nutrient utilised by the brain for energy production. One can see the reason for the depletion of our motor energy and the condition of hypoglycemia (which consequently leads to diabetes). Refined carbohydrates rapidly raise the blood sugar level, stimulating the pancreas to over-secrete insulin. This excess insulin removes too much sugar from the blood causing abnormally low blood sugar levels. In the normal digestive process, insulin allows for almost all the body's glucose absorbed after a meal to be stored by the liver in the form of glycogen. Glycogen is then converted to glucose and released into the blood between meals to maintain normal blood glucose concentrations.

Phosphorus, needed to build healthy bones, also plays an important part in energy conversions and storage in the body. It secretes the enzyme, phosphorlase, found in the liver and kidneys, to break down glycogen into glucose. Refined sugar depletes the body's supply of phosphorus in the body fluids with the over production of insulin. Because calcium needs to bind with phosphate and citrates for its transport to the bones, structural tissue and the nervous system, it cannot do so, because for calcium to be transported through the blood it must bind to protein.

The ingestion of refined carbohydrates – instead of fruits and vegetables – inhibits the digestion of protein, by not allowing for the liberation of sufficient acidity. This increases uric acid – acidosis – which causes phosphorus to be excreted in the urine along with calcium, "by a ratio of 1 : 2". The lower the calcium levels in the blood the weaker the enzymes will be. Protein deficiency in the blood reduces the function of the endocrine gland.

When there is insufficient phosphorus available, the insulin will promote the conversion of excess glucose in the liver into fatty acids to be transported and deposited as fat in connective tissues; this leads to obesity. The body then depends primarily on the metabolism of fat to supply its energy requirements, which also takes place mostly during starvation diets. And where there is not a relatively high blood glucose concentrate, there is the onset of diabetes.

CLASSIFICATION OF THE VITAL BODILY TEMPERAMENT

Whereas the vital bodily temperament remains part and parcel of all human beings, according to phrenology, its decided predominance (see Appendix for number interpretation) of the vital function in some individuals is accompanied by: a round head, well developed in the base; generally large organs of animal propensities; a rapid widening of the head from the corners of the eyes to the tip of the ears; side of the head well filled out; a full, broad rather than high forehead. Those so dispositioned, Fowler asserts:

> 7 Are fleshy; short and broad built; stocky; deep and large chested; broad and round shouldered; impetuous; impulsive; enthusiastic; hearty; good livers; fond of meats, condiments, stimulants, and animal pleasures; have a strong, steady pulse; large lungs and nostril; florid complexion; flushed face; sound and well set of teeth; great endurance of fatigue, privation and exposure; great love of fresh air, out-of-door exercise, and physical action, but not of hard work;

a restlessness which cannot endure in-door confinement, but must be out, and constantly doing something; great zeal, ardor of desire, and more practical common sense than book-learning; more general knowledge of people and things than accurate scientific attainment; more shrewdness and off-hand talent than depth; more availability than profundity; and love of pleasure than power of thought.

6 Are like 7, though not in as great extremes; generally fleshy and of good size and height, if not large; well-proportioned; broad-shouldered; muscular; prominent and strong-marked in features; coarse and homely; stern and harsh; strong but often awkward, and seldom polished; best adapted to some laborious occupation, and enjoy hard work more than books or literary pursuits; have great power of feeling, which requires much self-government; possess more talent than can exhibit to others; manifest mind more in business, in creating resources and managing matters, than in literary pursuits, or mind as such; prefer some light, stirring, active business, but dislike drudgery; turn everything, especially bargains, to good account; look out for self; get a full share of what is to be had; feel and act out "every man for himself," and are selfish enough, yet abound in good feeling; incline to become agents, overseers, captains, hotel-managers, butchers, traders, speculators, *etc.*, rather than anything requiring hard work – and are usually healthy, yet very sick when attacked, brought at once to crisis, and predisposed to gout, fevers, apoplexy, congestion of the brain *etc.*

5 Have a good share of life-force, yet none to spare; withstand a good deal, yet must not waste vitality, and should live in a way to improve it.

4 Have sufficient vitality to sustain life, and impart a fair share of energy to the functions, but by no means sufficient to expend full power, and should make its culture a first life-object.

3 Are rather weakly or feeble; often half prostrated by a feeling of exhaustion and lethargy; can keep doing all the time if slow, and careful not to overdo, the liability to which is great when activity is heightened; need much rest; cannot half work, or enjoy either body or mind; suffer much from fatigue and weariness, and would be glad to do, but hardly feel able.

2 Are too weak and low to be able to do, enjoy, or accomplish much; should both give the vital organs every possible facility for action, and also conserve every item of vitality; be extremely careful not to overwork, and spend much time in listless, luxuriating ease, while nature restores the wanting vitality.

1 Are almost dead form sheer inanition, that is, exhaustion from lack of nourishment.

TO CULTIVATE — Ascertain which of the vital organs is deficient, and take all possible pains to improve its action; see direction for increasing the action of the heart, lungs, stomach, *etc.*; alternate with rest and exercise; do away with melancholy, banish sadness, trouble, and all gloomy associations, and cultivate buoyancy and light-hearted-ness; enjoy the present, and make life a glorious holiday instead of a weary drudgery; if engaged in confining business, break up the monotony by taking a long leave of absence — a trip to the [Bay of Fundy], the [Caribbean], anywhere abroad, a long journey, by horticulture, or parties, or frolicking with children; by going into young and lively society, and exercising the affections; bringing about as great a change as possible in all your habits and associations. Especially cultivate a love of everything beautiful and lovely in nature, as well as study her philosophies; bear patiently what you must, but enjoy all you can; keep doing all you are able, but other things than previously, and what interest you. You should watch and follow your intuitions or instincts and if you feel a special craving for any special food or pleasure, indulge it. Be especially regular in sleep, exercise, eating, and all the vital functions, as well as be temperate in all things. Above all, keep your mind toned up to sustain the body. Aid your weak organs with will power, that is, bring a strong will to aid digestion, breathing *etc.*, and maintain that balance. Determine that you will *not* give up to weakness or death, but will live on and keep doing in *spite* of debility and disease. Fight life's battles like a true hero or heroine, and keep the head cool at all times by constantly altering the temperament with diet; the feet warm by exercise; the pores and evacuations open to cleansing and laxative foods; and heart warm by cherishing a love of life and its pleasures. And do not fail to keep up a gentle pounding and frequent brisk rubbing of the chest, abdomen, and feet, so as to start the mechanical action of the visceral (internal) organs. Nothing equals this for reviving dormant or exhausted vitality, and no one is too poor or can afford to be too occupied to benefit themselves in this manner.

TO RESTRAIN — The body must be fed well, but not to excess; never make a "god" of food. Those who manufacture vitality faster than they expend it, are large in the abdomen; too corpulent (fleshy); even obese; often oppressed for breath; surcharged with organic material; too sluggish to expend vitality as fast as it accumulates, and should therefore work, work, work, early and late, and with all their might, and as much as possible with their might, and as much as possible with their muscles and out-door; should eat sparingly, and of simple food; avoid rich gravies, butter, sweets, fats and pastry, instead live on fruits; sleep little; keep all the excretory organs free and open by high fibre diet, and especially the skin by frequent baths, the hot bath *etc.*; breathe abundantly, in order to burn up the surplus carbon; sit little, walk much; never yield to indolence; work up energy by hands and head, business and pleasure, any way, every way, but keep consuming vitality as fast as possible. Some fleshy persons, especially females, give up habitual idleness and folly; get "the blues", and lounge in a rocking-chair and bed. What is wanted to do, is not loiter around. Inertia is your cancer, and action is your cure. It flushed, feverish, nervous *etc.*, be careful not to overdo, and rely on air, warm bath, and gentle but continued exercise, active and passive, but not on remedies.

When the Creator said: "Let there be Light", the after-effect was impelled motion. Hence, motion remains the commandment for everything that lies in Creation. It is the most necessary and integral part of life. Without motion we could not walk, work or move – not to mention breathe, digest, or circulate blood; functions which are but action in its various phases.

THE LAW OF CONTINUOUS MOTION

Action is affected by means of bones and muscles or fibres, the fleshy portions of the system. These bones constitute the foundation on which the muscular superstructure is built, and are articulated at their ends by joints, and firmly bound together by ligaments which allow free motion. Toward the middle of these bones, the muscles are firmly attached, so that when they contract they give motion to the end of the bone opposite the belly of the muscle. These muscles, of which there are some 527 in the human body, constitute the lean meat or red flesh of all animals, and are rendered red by the immense number of minute blood-vessels which are ramified upon every fibre of every muscle, in order to re-supply that vital power expended by exercise. The contractile power of these muscles is truly astonishing, as is evident from the wonderful feats of strength and agility of which humans are capable, even though these muscles act under a great mechanical disadvantage.

Of critical importance is muscular exercise for the health of the lymphatic system, indispensable as it is to greatness and happiness. However, all parts must be exercised in proportionately if the whole is to be served. When the brain is worked more than the muscles, it becomes partially congested, loses its snap, leaves the mind dull, memory indefinite, and thoughts obtuse. One dare not aspire to greatness, however splendid their intellectual brain, without much vigorous exercise and real hard work. All eminent men and women had laid this foundation for their youth, and continue to exercise daily through life; while those students brought up without labor rarely take a prominent place in society, except in parrot-like scholarships. They always lack vim, polish and firmness of thoughts. And this deficiency grows as they age.

Take the life of John Quincy, for example, he was said to rise before the sun to take his exercise, and as he became old took much of it in swimming, which he said gave him the required exercise without heating his blood. Washington, was a hard-working farmer and soldier. Joan of Arc, the prodigy of feminine heroine - pictured as a young girl holding a pennon in her right hand, with her left on the hilt of he sword - gained her prominent place in history in the sphere of action. Clear about her calling - to throw the English out of France and bring the Dauphin Charles VII to his throne - pursued such with the fiercest bravery and innermost conviction, in the face of terrible ordeals. This decisive power of the feminine is dispensed from the goddess Pallas Athene (Minerra), of the ancient peoples, portrayed as a valiant being, with helmet, shield and spear. Her working is unflinching and unshakable, distinguished by sharp-eyed vigilance, reliability and conscientiousness. She defends, protects and sustains the motherland, and as "goddess of war" she accompanies armies.

A distinguishable character can only be gained in the sphere of action. A life full of work with real purpose; otherwise, in the Law of Necessary Movement, only the physical benefits, not the spirit, which consequently stands still. If spirit and body do not swing in harmony in one's activity, the latter will not be maintained and strengthened through its work, but become worn and exhausted through growing tension, from not receiving the spiritual strength it needs through the mediation of the animistic faculties. The stagnation of the spirit hampers the full development of the body. Consequently, the body in its own action must consume itself, causing it to wither and decay. It can no longer regenerate because the source for this - the spiritual – is lacking.

Psychotherapists are becoming more and more aware that the main cause of tension in the body is rooted in the subconscious, in the repressed intuitive brain. And, a regeneration can only begin there. Yet nothing extraordinary needs to be performed, if we set out to fulfil the purpose of our existence in the right manner. It is the nature of our *life's work and purpose* which predetermines the body-form, its further development linked to the design and function of the nervous system. We should not allow ourselves to be influenced by the marketing hype for the multitude of stimulants to add to our nourishment in order to energise our bodies. The right activity is the stimulant we need, that which gives us joy and fulfilment.

Then there are those high performance exercise gyms and sports clubs luring us with the promise of finely carved bodies, whether or not we genetically conform to such shapes. Extravagant physical activity only diverts the generative power through the wrong channels, and fitters it away uselessly in pursuit of personal satisfaction.

For some, their life's purpose is only athletic ambition, for it goes with self-exaltation and the delusion which comes with it that they are accomplishing something great. At times, even causing physical injury, which hinders any healthy progress and all the possibilities which have been provided for each of us in life. But the course of the strong currents of the spirit is meant to bring personal maturity for the benefits of the-world-at large and when blocked, act as hindrance to this purpose. In the end comes the "burnt-out syndrome", they fall ill, and eventually self-destruct. All due to our incapacity to comprehend that only through simplicity does the spirit develops inner strength from which the body derives its strength.

TO CULTIVATE: Take all the muscular exercise you can well endure but only gently; make yourself comfortably tired every day; choose those kinds of exercise most agreeable, but practice some kind assiduously; dance more and sit less.

TO RESTRAIN: Use the muscles less and the brain more.

THE MOTIVE CIRCULATORY SYSTEM

For the motive temperament, the lymphatic is the circulatory system, which is just as important as the cardiovascular and nervous systems and are closely linked.

The Lymphatic System

Unlike the heart, the lymphatic system is not pumped along, it function depends on muscular manipulation. Here lies a vast network of open-ended capillaries which permeate the body and are connected to three main filtering organs – the tonsils, spleen (the same size as the heart), and the thymus gland, which produces white blood cells (lymphocytes) vital to the immune system.

As well as playing a role in the body's defense mechanism, the lymphatic system is regarded as the transport system of the body. Its role involves the distribution of fluids and nutrients throughout the body. It also ensures that excess fluid and proteins are drained off so that the tissues do not swell. It ensures that fats, cell debris, foreign bodies, bacteria and products of metabolism are carried away.

Its gigantic network of capillaries transport lymph, about 18% of the body fluids (containing plasma proteins, foreign substances, and bacteria) which fills the spaces between the cells. The lymph capillaries flow one-way, slowly migrating lymph through the thoriac duct (one of the two main trunks of the lymphatic system, receiving lymph from both legs, the lower abdomen, left thorax, left side of the head, the left arm, and drains it into the left "short" artery passing upward to the right neck joint, or sternoclavicular) and from there reach the systemic blood circulation, at about three quarts per twenty four hours. They circulate to the intestinal mucosa and the bronchial mucosa and may also recirculate to mucosal sites in a lactating breast.

Of special significance in this transport are the small nodes, more than 100 pea or bean-sized organs which interrupt the pathway of the lymph vessels. These lymph nodes act as the filtering station. They filter and destroy micro-organisms and toxic substances. When there is an infection, the lymph nodes may swell, and what is treated as mere sore throat or ear infection is a reaction to antigens, simple glycoproteins invading bodily fluids. This invasion stimulates lymphocytes of the mucosa-associated lymphoid tissue from the intestinal duct (lumen) as well as from the blood component to react. In defense, antigen reactive B-cells migrate as lymphoblasts to the mesenteric (abdominal cavity) lymph nodes to mature. Once they become plasmablasts they begin their defensive journey through the system.

After stimulation and activation, B-cells develop into plasma cells with the specialised ability to copulate with and modify antigen to produce specific antibodies – lymphocytes (lymphocytic protease) – a specific one for each invading antigen, to neutralise possible harmful effects. These antibodies, with protolytic enzymes bound on the surface of their cell membrane, are similar to those found in large quantities in the lining of the gut that cover and protect the mucous membrane and control the absorption of antigens, bacterial and other toxins, pollen, from the intestinal lumen. These lymphocytic proteases have an increased affinity for infected cells due to their presence of foreign proteins in the cell membrane. In fact, protease actually break down the simple glycoproteins (toxins), rendering them ineffective, sparing the immune system from this task.

If these antibodies are not rejected into the intestinal duct with the outer layer of the intestinal tissue to be eliminated through the urinary tract, colon, skin and lungs, they may function like suppressor cells (which have the same effect as antibiotics). This may lead to a cytotoxic (destructive) immune reaction, such as cancer of the gut, Crohn's disease, colitis and celiac disease, and the various autoimmune diseases affecting the motive bodily temperament. For this reason it becomes imperative to support immune function by using biological remedies to help restore the bacterial colony back to normal by ensuring adequate elimination.

Refined Carbohydrates – Their Effects on the Motive Temperament

Glycoprotein, also called glycosylated protein, is a compound formed by the gut in the binding of protein with a carbohydrate. Certain enzymes, hormones, and antigens are glycoproteins. A diet too high in carbohydrates, causes excess glucose to bind to protein, giving rise to simple glycoproteins. This causes cell malignancy, hence autoimmune diseases, e.g., leukemia, arthritis, bursitis, and cancer.

AUTOIMMUNE DISEASES

As mentioned earlier, the ingestion of refined carbohydrates instead of fruits and vegetables, inhibits the digestion of protein. This allows for putrefaction in the gut, giving rise to bacteria, viruses and toxins. Intestinal bacteria, especially, increase in active and passive absorption of antigens and cause excessive strain on the gut associated with the immune system. Though it is the duty of the lymph to ensure that these antigens are carried away as waste, when there is an over abundance, they usually get deposited in the connective tissue.

The primary function of the gastrointestinal epithelium is to separate the luminal (sac-like) contents from the underlying mucosal fluids. The result is proper absorption of nutrients and the rejection of the toxic substances. The mucus lining of the gut, which naturally has a soft skin-like lining, consists mainly of a compound of proteins and carbohydrates to trap viruses, bacteria and toxins, as well as the protect the stomach lining from the highly acid gastric juice.

Too many simple sugars in the diet not only encourage high acidity, but poor absorption with the excess sugar joining proteins to form glycoproteins (antigens) which increase fructosamine levels, set to start cellular dysfunction and cellular structural damage. To compensate, the production of mucus increases to prevent damage, if possible, to the stomach lining from excess acid and antigens. However, too much mucus in the gut erects too much of a barrier between disaccharides (sucrase, maltase and lactase which permeate the intestinal mucosal wall for completing digestion) and complex carbohydrates (polysaccharides starch). This prevents healthy digestion, because the alkaline pancreatic amylase cannot adequately break down polysaccharides into disaccharides to be absorbed by the liver for its synthesis to glycogen, on which the brain relies for its fuel.

Neither will there be adequate production of lactic acid from lactase to stabilise the pH in the small and large intestines which is vital for creating an environment for healthy intestinal flora. The result is a disturbed acid coating which allows for the attack of pathogenic micro-organisms and environmental toxins. Moreover, lactic acid is a natural substance that activates cell regeneration whereby it raises respiration of malignant cells, to activate the healing process. Hence the "viscous cycle":

- altered and improper sugar digestion, leads to excess sugar joining proteins to form glycosylated proteins, which increases fructosamine levels and results in cellular dysfunction and structural damage.
- lack of proper starch digestion results in malabsorption, fatigue, infection, inflammation, and likely poor protein assimilation, hence catabolic states, *i.e.*, high body fat – sign of the body eating itself, its muscles.
- poor digestion increases production of insulin, negative production of prostaglandins (one of the hormone-like fluids found in the womb, brain, kidneys, semen, *etc.*), abnormal cell divisions, and secondary lowering of glucagon (a hormone produced by the pancreas that raises blood sugar levels – the opposite effect of insulin).
- canabolic (cytotoxic) states, the destruction of cells – bursitis, rheumatoid arthritis, *etc.*, – pro-inflammatory conditions results which cause excessive stimulation to the endocrine, pancrine, and autocrine system.
- pro-inflammatory response from diet causes most cells to degranulate (degenerate) in the synovial tissue and cause a pathological response.

Cystic Fibrosis

Cystic fibrosis is overproduction of mucus in the gut, which obstructs the intestinal glands; of the pancreas, depleted alkaline pancreatic amylase enzymes; of the bronchi, bronchiolitis. A diet high in simple carbohydrates or one who is sugar intolerant experiences the state of acidosis, wherein the body must produce excess mucus to protect the respective membranes.

Thrombosis

In the synovial fluid around the joints, and the vitereous and humors of the eyes is found hyaluronic acid – a component of mucopolysaccharide (of the complex carbohydrates) and proteins. This acid acts as a binding and protective agent of the ground substance of connective tissue.

Hyaluronic acid is also found in heparin (anticoagulant factor) produced in the liver cells, some white blood cells, and certain sites, and acts like an enzyme to inhibit the enzyme thrombin (coagulation factor) from synthesising protein in the final stage to coagulate the blood. The final product of blood coagulation process is the microbal molecule called fibrin *mononer*, which links with similar molecules to weave a fibrous mesh that forms the basis of a blood clot (thrombus), used to seal off damaged tissues and prevent the migration of disease-causing agents or toxins to other areas of the body. During the repairing process, serum protolytic enzymes called plasmins, begin to break down the fibrin into smaller, soluble peptides and amino acids.

Thrombosis is the condition where, in the oxidation process, insufficient protolytic activity of blood plasma in the vessels increases the production of fibrin into the fungus thrombozyte, which obstructs blood flow to the tissue, hence the condition called hyperemia; if this occurs in the artery to the brain it can lead to stroke; in the artery supplying the heart, heart attacks; in the veins it releases histamine, serotonin and negative prostaglandins (muscle contracting hormone), which causes inflammatory pain. But not without first exhausting the adrenals and the nervous system or unbalancing the hormones which must react to the harmful agent, thereby threatening the lymphatic system (lymhotasis). Apart from a complete stoppage of circulation to the affected area and a delay of the phagocytic stage of inflammation, scar tissue forms due to delayed healing.

Protein produces fibrin, as well as antibodies, and phagocytic enzymes (including many white blood cells), all part of the body's defense mechanism. Therefore, it needs to be properly digested and utilised by the body, not only to bind free calcium in the blood to support the structural tissue and nervous system, but to prevent and eliminate blood clots, and accompanying hypercalcemania (abnormally high presence of calcium in the blood) and/or hypercalcuria (in the urine). This cannot happen when one's diet is high in refined carbohydrates.

A link, then, connects the disease thrombosis and glycoproteins. The imbalance between the number of fibrin clots formed and the amount of plasmin present to dissolve the clot, can be traced back to the overindulgence in refined carbohydrates. Such a diet not only depletes essential nutrients, especially B vitamins, and impairs the conversion of carbohydrates to energy, but fat and protein metabolism as well. Suppressed protolytic enzyme activity prevents the cleaving of glucose for metabolism and leaves too much protein in the tissue (excess alkaline reserves), resulting in the overproduction of fibrin (thrombozytes), which if not dissolved, apart from the above mentioned conditions, can also lead to irreparable DNA damage – osteoporosis, osteoarthritis, degenerative disc problems, bone spurs *etc.*

CLASSIFICATION OF THE MOTIVE BODILY TEMPERAMENT

The bones and muscles collectively constitute the framework of the body – give it its build and form – and are to humans what the timbers, ropes, and pulleys are to the ship, and constitute the motive temperament. Though part and parcel of all human body frame, its predominance (see Appendix for number interpretation) in some individuals confers power of *constitution*, and of strength and character and feeling. According to Fowler these individuals are:

> 7 Are lean, spare; of good size and height, and athletic; have strongly marked features; large nose; high and large cheek bones; large and broad front teeth; all the bones projecting; a deep, grum, bass voice; distinctly marked muscles and blood-vessels; large joints; hard flesh; great muscular power or physical strength; ease of action, and love of physical labor, of lifting, working *etc.*; dark and often coarse,

stiff, abundant, and perhaps bushy hair; if a man, a black and heavy beard; dark skin and eyes; a harsh, expressive visage; strong but coarse and harsh feelings – the movements like those of the draught-horse, slow but powerful and efficient; tough; thorough-going; forcible; strong marked, if not idiosyncratic; determined, and impressive both physically and mentally; and stamp your character on all you touch. With motive 7, mental 6, and vital 5, you are capable of power and sustained mental effort, and great power in any department, swaying a commanding influence over mankind, taking lead in a large business. This temperament is always accompanied by prodigious coronal and perceptive powers, firmness, and combativeness – its natural accompaniment – the very organs required to re-increase its force and efficiency, and indispensable to its exercise.

6 Are like the 7, except less in degree; are tough, hardy, and strong constitutioned; evince power, efficiency, and force in whatever is undertaken, use strong expressions; are stout, limber-jointed, and need and can endure a world of action and fatigue; are like a fire made of anthracite coal, making a slow but powerful and continuous heat, and will make a decided mark in the business world, or in whatever department these energies may be exercised. With the vital 6 or 7, and the mental 3 or 4, are broad and prominent in form; large, tall, well proportioned, broad-shouldered and muscular; usually coarse featured, homely, stern, and awkward; enjoy hard work more than books or literary pursuits; have great power of feeling, and thus require self-government; are endowed with good sense, but have a poor way of showing it; are strong-minded, but possess more talents than power to exhibit them; manifest talents more in managing machinery, creating resources, and directing large operations than in mind as such; improve with age, growing better and more intellectual; accomplish wonders; are hard to beat, indomitable, and usually useful citizens, but endowed with strong passions when roused; and capable of being deeply depraved, especially if given to drinking.

5 Have a good share of the hearty, enduring, efficient, and potential; more right forward, with determination and vigour, irrespective of hindrances; bring a good deal to pass; are like 6, only less so.

4 Are not deficient in motive power, yet more would be better; wrought up by special circumstances, can put forth unwonted strength; but it will be spasmodic, and liable to overstrain; can work hard, but are reluctant to; prefer the sedentary to the active, and business to labor; with the vital 6 or 7 are physically lazy and do only what cannot be avoided, and need to cultivate muscular power.

3 Dislike activity directed to some purpose or end; prefer to labor; may be quick and flashy, but more powerful; lack strength and weight of character; need much more exercise than they love to take; and first of all should cultivate both muscular action and strength of character. With a vital 6, and mental 6 or 7, are rather small-boned, but plump, well formed, light complexioned, and often handsome; have unusually auburn or flaxen hair; are most exquisitely organised, most pathetic and sympathetic, sentimental, exalted, and spiritual; have redoubled glow and fervor of feeling, derived from both the vital and the mental, which they are hardly able to contain; easily receive and communicate impressions; are quite too much influenced by impression; are fond of company, if not forward in it; have a quick, clear, sharp, keen, active mind, and good business talents; a ready flow of ideas and a talent for communicating them, either on paper or in social conversation; show taste, refinement, and delicacy in everything; have an under-current of pure, virtuous feeling, which will prevent the grosser manifestation of animal passion, and give the intellectual and moral ascendency; sin only under sudden and powerful excitement; are passionately fond of poetry, novels, tales, light and sentimental reading, belles-lettres, newspaper, *etc.*, and inclined to attempt

this kind of composition; have a retentive memory, shrewdness, smartness, and enough of the selfishness to take good care of self, yet not sufficient momentum or power to become great, but rather effeminate. This temperament is found much more often and more perfect in females than males.

Children thus organised are precocious, and liable to die prematurely. Mental 7, vital 5, and motive 3, may be smart, but cannot be great; may be brilliant, but are flashy, meteoric, vapid, too emotional, imaginative, and impulsive, and like a fire made of pine wood or shavings, intense, but momentary.

2 and 1 Work, walk, move, and use muscles only when obliged to; pre-inclined much more to the emotional and vapid than potential, and should cultivate the muscles assiduously.

The mental bodily temperament embraces the brain and the nerves, or that portion of the system called into exercise in the production of the conscious mind as such, of thought-volition, feeling, sensation, memory, Whereas the former two temperament perform the mechanical actions and work of the physical body, the mental is actually what "leads" in these things, to that which is willed by the spirit and which the brain and the bodily implements then enact.

THE AUTONOMIC NERVOUS SYSTEM

To gain a deeper understanding of the mental temperament is to do so in relation to the autonomic nervous system. Like Pavlov believed, the higher nervous activity determines externally realised behavior and is a function of the brain; he cites the differences in psychology and behavior that were also found in the fine details of the brain's activity – the flow pattern of the human temperament, controlled by nerves centres in the spinal cord and brain stem and fine-tuned by the intuitive brain.

The nervous system is divided into two aspects: (1) the somatic movement, allowing voluntary control over the skeletal muscles of the head, limbs and body and (2) the autonomic movement, the involuntary movement and control of the cardiac and smooth muscles. Ideally, this homeostasis is kept between the sympathetic branch or 'interceptive-tonic' patterns and the parasympathetic branch or 'exteroceptive-phasic' influences. Each organ and gland is primarily stimulated by one of the automatic nervous system's two branches - either the sympathetic or the parasympathetic. Generally, the sympathetic branch accelerates organ functions while the parasympathetic acts as a decelerator, the two branches exerting opposing effects.

The sympathetic (tonic) branch connects to the central nervous system by fine branches linking each ganglion with the spinal cord. Its nerves are distributed to the blood vessels, sweat glands, salivary glands, heart, lungs, intestines and other abdominal organs, and the genitals. This branch forms the basis for the exteroceptive-phasic influences, the going out of the materialised impressions which have already come through in the astral body (thought-form). It not only responds to the transmissions of spiritual impressions and intuitive volition with such reactions as colours, sounds, attraction or repulsion, but also to emergencies and sudden environmental changes initiating stress which acts upon the immune system via the aura.

Its tonic (involuntary or fluid) reactions govern postures, often termed 'Postural Reactions'. However, the postural fluid can degenerate through continual stress, progressive disease or prolonged mental pressure, causing us to become rigid and rather stereotyped in our response to stimuli.

The sympathetic branch tends to respond as a whole, particularly during emergencies or sudden environmental changes which initiate stress. Stressful experiences such as pain, evoke what is termed the "Fight or Flight" reaction, the built-in mechanism to prepare us to act in stressful situations. This nerve branch is more enduring and secretes adrenocortitrophic hormone (adrenaline) of the pituitary, followed by increased activity of the adrenal cortex which diffuses adjustment calculated to maintain a continuity in the organism's conduct, by serving as a 'substratum' (enzymatic function) for the parasympathetic branches.

If this reaction is ongoing whether by stress, anxiety or irritation to the viscus of the phrenic nerve, the adrenal becomes exhausted. We become predisposed toward the sympathetic branch (the emotional or astral plane) of the autonomic nervous system. This increases the consumption of oxygen causing the diaphragm and other respiratory muscles to lock into an "exhalation mode". That is, the condition where there is an exaggerated expulsion of carbon dioxide in the extracellular fluid which causes the continuous release of an acid called acetylcholine and the blood becomes alkaline. Over an extended period of time this pushes the entire body to a state of alkalosis or hyperventilation.

Fortunately, however, after relaying a nerve impulse, the enzyme cholineterase rapidly destroys the acetycholine released during the transmission of the nerve so that subsequent impulses do not pass. However, if the action of acetycholine is blocked, it causes muscular paralysis.

The parasympathetic branch leads from the brain to the lower spinal cord. It is responsible for those quick and localised movements of head limbs and body, caused by nerve impulses arising in the motor area of the brain and cranial nerves and by nerves emerging from the spinal cord to connect with the skeletal muscles. These phasic reactions come and go. The parasympathetic branch supplies nerves to such organs as the rectum, bladder and genitals. In conjunction with its compliment – the sympathetic nervous branch – it controls or decelerates the involuntary body movement, such as the intestinal movements, beating of the heart, sweat, salivation, Hence it offers only a temporary readjustment to a momentary type of situation.

A predisposition towards the parasympathetic (thinking) branch, with stimuli upon the phrenic nerve, can lock one in an "inhalation mode". When this happens there is an inability to expel adequate amounts of carbon dioxide which causes its excessive accumulation in the extracellular fluid, acidifying the blood. Over an extended period, the body is pushed toward a state of respiratory acidosis or hypoventilation; decelerated heart contractions and lowered blood pressure; and accelerates the digestive process.

THE CENTRAL NERVOUS SYSTEM

Of critical importance in this intercourse is the overall health of the central nervous system (with its seven energy centres or intermediary points, also called *chakras,* relating also to the seven states of conscious development). Its main impulse centre has its basis in the spiritual connection to the astral body in the area of the solar plexus, the gut; the others are found at areas around the base of the spine, the lower belly, the heart, throat, brow and crown. Through the medium of the spinal column, and by means of the nerves which go off from the spinal marrow through the joints of the back-bone, the brain holds intercourse with every other part of the body. The nerves are so ramified upon every portion of its surface that not even a needle can penetrate any portion of it without lacerating them, thus producing pain.

The spinal marrow is composed of four principal columns, the two anterior ones exercising voluntary motion, the two posterior ones for sensation. If the nerves leaving the root of the two posterior columns are severed, the parts on which they are ramified will be destitute of sensation, without feeling, though one remains able to move. On severing the nerves which go off from the two anterior columns, one will feel the prick of a needle, but not be able to move the limbs along which the nerve travels. Hence the two anterior or motor columns are in direct connection with the sympathetic branch leading back brain, which gives rise to the movements of the body, and accordingly the skin and adjacent flesh is the seat of much more intense pain from wounds than the internal portions.

The aerial-like nerve receptor and transformer of the intellectual brain completes the physically visible reactions of walking, sitting, talking, *etc.*, through the two anterior or motor columns. It is the antenna of the (unconscious) mind which excites the tonic invisible movements which can only be felt: movements such as heat or cold, colours, sounds, attraction or repulsion, as well as heaviness or lightness. These invisible movements produce an equivalent effect in the conscious brain which subsequently becomes strongly perceptible in the feelings of the entire body – the phasic reaction. Hence the impulses of the intuitive brain form the basic ground on which the conscious brain devolves. The interceptive impulses of the conscious mind do not merely sustain them, they also restrain them and determine their effectiveness, in other words, decelerate them.

And so it is for our everyday experiences. If it was not for the receptive and transmissive activity of the sympathetic nervous system, the absorption of impressions for what we experience could not happen. This influence upon the nervous system holds true for all experiences. When that which is to be experienced can also be an excitation upon feeling, be it impulses within or influences from outside, from which we may experience emotions of either happiness or sadness.

To experience life that surrounds us in Nature, for example, a flower, the stimulated sympathetic nervous system adjusts itself to remain open for the image to fall upon the retina, stimulating the necessary impulses of the cortex (the area of the third eye chakra) and radiating other bodily nerves. This in turn stimulates the imagination, generating feelings. We absorb the nature of the feeling and send it to be assimilated by the intuitive back-brain, in order to exercise from there a corresponding pressure on the nerve centre in the solar plexus region; this then sends the picture back to the frontal brain as comprehension, from having aroused an intuitive perception in accordance with feeling.

The sequences, however, take place at the speed of lightening. In the case of the flower - colours, fragrance and all that is in one's capacity to absorb. The same goes for the understanding of the behavior of others in our surroundings, although the actual experience may only be understood or grasped long after the act itself, based on the receptivity of the nervous system.

It must be understood, that the nervous system does not and cannot operate simultaneously between the two operations – the sympathetic and the parasympathetic nerve branches – between reception and transmission, in the normal course of activity. It is subject to only one state at a time, either the activity of the spirit or the intellect. However, bearing higher spirit-seed within, we unite the ethereal beyond (the world of picture or form) and the dense material of this world (the intellect), and it becomes possible for us to survey and experience both simultaneously.

THE MENTAL CIRCULATORY SYSTEM

Nerve impulses circulate the mental temperament, and are important as the cardiovascular and lymphatic systems.
The human central nervous system can be likened to a train at a terminus with irremovable lines connected to intermediary stations. The train lines are like nerve branches spreading throughout the organism, along which external stimulus and volitional desires roll according to the position of stations and curves. These intermediary nerve points of the body are represented by the seven endocrine glands, organs and body system: the pineal gland; the pituitary gland, eyes, ears; the thyroid gland, respiratory system; the thymus gland, circulatory system; the pancreas, digestive system; the gonads, reproductive system; the adrenal glands and kidneys.

Temperament drives the nervous system. When an impulse comes in, the nervous system, like the train engine, is animated, depending on the nature of the individual's temperament. The speed of the train – the temperament, offering a pleasant or unpleasant ride – likened to the pace of one's life, is the key to the overall health or disease, mental stability or instability of the organism. The speed, whether impetuous (excitable), quiet unvarying (temperate), too slow, or variations of these, is determined by the state of the nervous system from which action is performed.

Over-excitable, immoderate types develop high-strung nervous systems. This type is more or less driven and affected by external forces and happenings. They thrive on impulses and act on spontaneity. Egoism is their greatest sin, in their every act they demand full attention of those around. For this reason they assume more responsibility than they are able to accomplish, which creates a sense of guilt, anxiety and despair if things do not go right. But they are easily distracted and their thoughts stray easily, and unless they compel themselves to accomplish a task they tend to develop only enough steam to start, not enough to finish. Failure to channel creative energy to constructive end create their poor self-image; this is why they always need others.

Hence their self-destructive lifestyles and accompanying defective manner of eating; the result of anxiety syndrome, characterised by any of the following symptoms: hysteria; tension without cause; irritable or angry response to stimuli or frustration; obsessive fears and hypochondria; fear of social activities; indecisiveness associated with suspiciousness; inattention and failure to recall; difficulty falling asleep; nightmares; despondency and pessimism; fatigue; appetite impairment; faintness; and or bouts similar to vertigo (altered consciousness).

Weak types, those who repress their emotions, suffer depressed anxiety and melancholia. The weakening of their volitional desires heightens the sensitivity and irritability of their nervous system. Their inability to satisfy the self-preserving instincts (love, boldness, sternness, food and drink, self-control, ambition, self-respect, independence) sinks them deep into melancholic depression, because their developmental needs were not met. This altered spiritual movement, the depression of the vital force, is called *neurasthesia;* those who inhibit their emotions, rarely express them in thoughts, words or action. They are usually too fearful and cautious to try anything new or different, lacking the vigilance to effect any change in their lives – to step out on a limb, so to speak; they lack self-confidence and are easily confused when it comes to decision making. This disorder of their psychic and mental function leads to their neurotic behavior.

As said in the Introduction, Freeman observed how permanently fixated the postural substrate can become in one so inhibited, especially when some persistent motivational excitant is thwarted from attaining an adequate discharge. This postural fixation (repressed intuitive perception) he pointed out, "helps to explain the loss of contact with reality of many psychotic patients". And, external influence (mental stimulus) has little effect and no amount of persuasion will ever change this individual's outlook. Only the individual can turn his or her own life around at the level of soul, and only if the mental equilibrium has not already been seriously disturbed. This is what it means by changing the points.

These two nerve conditions are the extreme, however, with some individuals having mixtures of both, the limitless variety of intermediate reactions more common through an overlap. Where there is extreme imbalance in the temperament, one will find the sanguine and choleric types leaning more to the overexcitable, more so the sanguine; while the melancholic and the phlegmatic lean more to the inhibited. The phlegmatic is said to have the most stable nervous system of all. Then again, factors such as the region of one's birth; race; stellar and ground radiations at any particular time; diet; the ageing process; but more than all, the maturity of one's soul, combine to affect temperament. One thing is clear, the unstable condition of the nervous system causes either anxiety syndrome, or neurotic behavior; whereby one yields to temperament instead of controlling it, developing conditions where one behaves like tyrant – to the self and society.

Over excitable types live, to a greater or lesser extent, not a rational, but an emotional life governed not by premeditated (cortical), but by unpremeditated (subcortical) activity. Premeditated activity has a definiteness of purpose, requiring deep reflection, orderliness, precision, thoroughness and organisational skill to achieve the desired result. Hence one can understand the occasional schizophrenic behavior and morbid imagination of the so-called perceptive types if the nervous system is unstable. The activity of the artist, for instance, is not of the frontal area of the brain (cerebrum), but of the intuitive back-brain. The opposite is the case for thinkers, it is predominantly in the frontal brain.

Unpremeditated Action (Mental health or ill-health)

Looking at unpremeditated action, must be done in two parts, for there are two kinds. One flares up on impulse and is already an act in only a few seconds. Such proceeds directly from the spirit by way of the intuitive brain to the physical organs. This becomes noticeable in moments of fear or anger – the "Flight or Fight" reaction, whereby powerful changes occur in the body causing the blood to run cold or agitate in rage. Here the tedious intellectual brain is eliminated, which otherwise would have to mediate the way of the will right up to the impression on the activity of the body. Here one is more or less robbed of their senses, standing "beside oneself", losing self-control and is responsible for their actions only to a limited extent.

The other kind flashes in the frontal brain, and belongs to the intellectual category. These are emotional disturbances or stimuli which influence the activity of the body. This runs from mild depression, to schizophrenia, to extreme cases where the individual is considered "possessed", which is, however, oftentimes mistaken for insanity.

Still, this exploration into unpremeditated action is unobjectionable if it takes place outside of the context of self-control, *i.e.*, the "letting go" of oneself. For it is the conscious suppression of the impulses of the intuitive perception, whether through overstimulation of the mental brain or inhibition of volitional desires of the soul, that establish imbalances in the brain. The result is an uncontrollable behavioral pattern, to the extreme involuntary or aimless movements, so-called pendulum movements. Through lack of self-control, the individual suppresses the spiritual-intuitive brain, oppressing and confining it till it becomes stifled.

Hence, conditions that usually start out depressions gradually evolve into one who can be classified as having delusions, or "possessed". One may only be "possessed" of a fixed idea but are otherwise normal, monomania. There are others who only have lucid hours or moments, and some who talk irrationally at times, in that the emotional body is connected to the organ of speech.

And when it is not the case where it is a stronger-willed individual that does the controlling, the extreme happens where the 'indolent-victim' provides a particular inferior blood-radiation which gives the opportunity to another "bodiless" human spirit (already departed life in the physical body) existing in the victim's surrounding, bearing malicious qualities to control the brain, periodically or perpetually. The stronger spirit forces its will in such a way that the rightful owner living within the body surrenders because they are either too weak or lazy to exercise the power of will, *i.e.*, to direct thought and feeling to the liberating effect. The possession causes a straining of the nerves of the brain, the limbic system, which is literally shaken up and thrown into confusion and causes the individual to act and talk irrationally at times. Yet the brain may be quite healthy, it is only the fight of the two different spirits which cause the confusion.

"Possession" happens to anyone irrespective of colour, class or creed. It is due to a weary or indolent spirit. It has nothing whatsoever to do with intellectual cleverness. An individual can be intellectually sharp and clever, and yet have a stifled spirit which allows an alien spirit to take total control of the physical body, even pushing out the soul, crowding it out with the exception of a small part which it cannot steal without endangering the life of the body itself. The alien spirit not only makes complete use of the brain, but also subjugates other parts of the body for itself and its purposes. Hence the split personalities we witness around us amongst family, friends and strangers, driving many disturbed ones to commit suicide over the way they have acted, or over their powerlessness to act. Still these individuals are not truly insane, they are only mentally disturbed and can be helped with therapy based on spiritual guidance supported by appropriate food and drink, to alter the blood radiation.

INSANITY

Insane are those within whom an imbalance in the brain is forcibly brought about by disease. Insanity is a physical disease. It can be caused by inflammation of the brain, giving rise to those mental derangements consequent of many fevers; by delirium tremens; by softening of the brain, weakening of mentality; and many similar phenomena. An imbalance may also be caused by brain injury, which may, for example, inflame the tune centre, causing a singing disposition, or the cautiousness centre, causing groundless fears. There is yet another group, classified as "morally insane" or depraved beyond reform, incorrigibles. Their intellect and moral sentiments are so underdeveloped and propensities so heavy (large), their baseness and passions sink their souls toward evil doing. These are society's hardened criminals, who nourish their propensities by continually indulging in dark deeds, they are servants of their instinct.

Propensity is defined as, a craving which verges on the intuition, on that which is spiritual, although only at its outermost edge. This becomes a burning desire and holds the spirit where it can obtain gratification to enjoy *inner sensations.*

Hence the words of Pavlov: "There are no special genes, for example, for humanism or alturism or genes for antisocial behavior. But there are genetically determined properties of the psyche [soul], the combination of which, when they are intertwined with certain social conditions, facilitates the person with either a high moral sense who feels a revulsion for criminal activity as well as careerism and greed, or it facilitates the development of a person who has little understanding of what morality is, with all the consequences that entails."[21]

MOODS AND EMOTIONS

The passions of moods and emotional swings are but the concentration of shallow and confused thinking, the hurrying together of thoughts. Such causes us to act hastily, which gives way to error, especially in our dealing with others.

Over-stimulation in the thought process is followed by an emotional drainage, "let down", for such a state cannot be sustained by the nerves. In so doing, the individual voluntarily opens the self, the emotional astral plane of light, to the possibility of unpleasant and sometimes harmful alien influences, even "bodiless spirits", developing changes in mood. Yet the one so affected is the one who wills this on the self and only a such one, in exercising the power of volition, can break this influence. It may also be broken by another who places such a one under his or her mesmeric healing power.

The same applies to artificially stimulating the imagination by reading, occult practices or some other means. Other than mental agitation this leads to phasic reactions as well, the body becomes enfeebled and the sympathetic nerve branch becomes overwrought - autonomic dysregulation.

The experience can also be that of seeing phantoms actually rushing at the individual, which are only forms created by one's imagination. Phantoms manifest as shadows which eventually fade as the weak thought-volition from which they are formed also fades. They are formed and sustained by one's fear and anxiety. Having no life of their own, phantoms are completely dependent upon the volitional desires of their authors who themselves are fearful human beings. Although methods of instilling concentration and courage are used to exorcise them, only fearlessness and courage of an inner composure can truly expel such astral forms in a natural manner.

Alongside mental ill-health is usually a pathological disease. Constantly sounding the body's alarm system – the "Fight or Flight" reaction accelerates organ function, which eventually starts organic changes due to overstimulation and a dominance of the sympathetic nerve branch. Their heart constantly palpitates and the blood pressure rises, with an increase in cellular metabolism which generally slows or shuts down their digestive process. The overstimulation of adrenocorticotrophic hormone of the pituitary also increases thyroid function. This usually leads to periods of overstimulation of the sexual organs and compulsive sexual desires.

Phasically, one finds the mucous membrane of the head region dry; the bronchial muscles relaxed, vascoconstriction of blood vessels and smooth muscles; sluggishness of bowels (constipation); reduced gastric hydrochloric acid (HCL) and pancreatic enzymes secretion; dilated pupils; decreased saliva production; relaxed gallbladder function; exhausted adrenals; reduced kidney output; decreased prostatic secretion; and/or contracted anal sphincter; *etc.* - symptoms heightening during periods of rest.

However, as already mentioned, health crisis – at intermediary nerve points and curves, which usually mark the precancerous phase of any disease or before a mental breakdown – is a sign to the train operator, to slow down when reaching such points (of organ and tissue degeneration), and then to stop and turn, to change the points. Slowing represents the act of personal reflection, stopping the decision taken by the individual, which one is always free to make until reaching the last opportunity to choose, to reverse symptoms.

This process of reflective action is what psychotherapists need to facilitate, in working to help restore and preserve one's mental dysfunction. An involvement wherein the subject engages in a process where he or she takes full responsibility in observance of the Natural Laws; not only in the principles of thought-form, but also that of nutrition which influences volitional desires (the spiritual) and action (the material); conscious of their full responsibility, cognisant they are independent in their basic decision.

The turning point is automatic, by restraint of the overdominant temperament or the cultivation of the same. It must be a self-conscious turn from one's self-destructive mode of living and accompanying defective manner of eating which attracts negative influences from outside, to support the propensity that could be genetically inherited or newly driven. Whatever the resolution, the inevitable end which in accordance with the immutable animistic laws of continuous development pervades the nervous system, leads more and more toward a definite goal conforming to one's attitude.

Just like the network of train lines, connected to the autonomic nerve branch are the sympathetic and parasympathetic nerve branches which one can use to change direction (predominance) and so reach the one first contemplated – homeostasis. Depending on which branch is predominant, turning the points occasionally by removing the stressful stimuli, one may remove intermediary blockages before tissue damage is irreversible. This, however, requires a disciplined holistic approach. Detecting such imbalances, slowing them, or arresting their development can be done using safe biological means (herbal, homeopathic, probiotics, and super food complexes, *etc.*).

Hence, a simultaneous increase in stimulation by the parasympathetic nervous system can help retard this sympathetic dominance. Apart from engaging in more mental activities which require using the rational mind more and the correct diet to buffer the alkalinity of the body fluids, there are also herbal remedies which have been clinically proven to directly affect the autonomic nervous system by enhancing the activity of the parasympathetic branch. One such herb is hawthorn which has the compound called acethycholine, said to "serve as a neurotranmitter of the effector cells located at the terminal nerve endings innervated by the parasympathetic nervous system. Its increased intake can stimulate the release of more transmitter molecules with each neuron firing, thus amplify signals from the neurons to the target cells they innervate. The result is an improvement in parasympathetic nerve transmission which can retard overstimulation of sympathetic nervous system ...."[22]

If the dominance leans towards the parasympathetic (thinking and feeling) nerve branch, that is, giving more to the rational with little or no emotion, the very rigid type emerges. With these individuals, the opposite occurs. An over-stimulation of the motive in this manner eventually leads to decreased heart contractions and low blood pressure, which generally speed the digestive process. Reduced adrenocorticophic hormone activity of the pituitary gives rise to sexual indifference, low libido, psychologically-based impotence; bladder tenemus; in females – anemia, dysmenorrhoea, mental instability with sedentary lifestyles; decreased thyroid activity; hypotensive, weak individuals, and exhaustion. Phasically, one experiences wet mucus membrane of the head region; contracted bronchial muscles; increased peristalsis and gastrointestinal motility giving rise to diarrhea; constricted pupils; increased salivation; inhibited gallbladder function; and relaxed anal sphincter – symptoms heightened during periods of activity.

In addition to balancing mental activity with artistic pursuits, regular Nature trips and, buffering excess acidity in the body fluid, the simultaneous increase of stimulation activating the sympathetic nervous system helps retard this parasympathetic dominance. Unsaturated fatty acid has been clinically proven to reverse parasympathetic dominance. The essential fatty acids, linoleic acid, linolenic acid and arachidonic acid are needed for the production of energy (ATP), which is used in the glandular secretion of hormones, conduction of nerve impulses and other functions influencing the autonomic nervous system. In addition, phospholipids, formed through fatty acid metabolism, are required for the synthesis of the myelin sheaths protecting nerve fibres. Fatty acids are necessary for glandular activity, especially the adrenals which are responsible for secreting the hormone epinephrine and norepinephrine in response to sympathetic nerves in all parts of the body and have the potential to counter symptoms of an overstimulated parasympathetic system.

So we can now see that many disorders are the direct result of this nerve imbalance in the brain equilibrium, due to ongoing bodily tension. The ability to handle these bodily tensions, culminated with the instability of today's stressful life causes ceaseless agitation which brings about this nervous and organic disorder of the stomach and intestines. Hence defective nutrition and the passage of microbes in the circulatory system, which depends on the organic health of the mental faculties.

The aura is the first to be affected by inner and outer stress. The weaker the aura, the less stress one can simply shrug off, and the less the immune system can respond to foreign invasion; whereby viruses and cancerous cells are allowed to freely proliferate.

Such disorders, however, are rare in circles where life is organised, simple and free of anxiety. This does not speak to those who seek a life of ease and comfort, away form themselves, from their self-centeredness, to find their way to others. But to those of an inner spiritual maturity, those who are able to maintain peace in the midst of turmoil. They are immune to nervous disorders. These are individuals who usually enjoy lasting success and prosperity as the natural consequence of their inner stability. Such comes on its own accord, a natural consequence of their deeds, as they are uplifted by the consequences of their own activities.

Therefore, only a healthy limbic system allows for the awakening of inner powers. The brain region involved are the *amygdala, hippocampal* and *hypothalamus*, their activities govern self-preservation of the species (*e.g.*, searching for food, fighting) and preservation of the species (*e.g.*, reproduction and care of offspring), the expression of fear, rage, and pleasure and the establishment of memory patterns. Only in its integrated state, can we perform our greatest achievements, thus be better able to transform this world and reverse the present course of society which appears so wrong. Giving birth to Paradise on Earth, where there would be no more immorality, shamelessness, bigotry, prejudice, disrespect – no form of debauchery. The ideal society of the future with love as its basis. Where everyone brings love into form in every moment of their existence and lets it be the purpose of their lives. We breathe love. Feel it. Create with and in it. For love is the breath of life, without it how can life be sustained?

Sleep and Dream States

The cerebrum is called the day brain, because it activates the intellect. In day-consciousness, *i.e.*, having the ability to think in waking state, the frontal brain performs the so-called hard labor. It transforms all impressions conveyed to it by the back brain, to become intelligible. For this reason alone the frontal brain grows weary and needs sleep.

While the frontal brain sleeps, the back brain, also called the dream brain, does not, neither does it have the need to share in this sleep, but to simply rest, to repose. We all have had the experience of merely resting the body while being awake, having no need to sleep.

While the frontal brain rests in the sleep the whole course of thinking also ceases. The inability to think, termed sleep, leaves the back brain in its self-conscious identity. The intuitive back brain is always awake. This gives rise to the dream state.

The dream state is the resulting activity of the intuitive brain, due to the influence of the spirit. In the right condition it is unaffected by internal or external influences, which allows for clear and unconfused dreams – only where there is a harmonious relation of the operations of the intuitive brain and the intellectual brain. In fact, we will no longer receive dreams but actual experiences of the spirit received and produced by the back brain while the frontal brain rests in sleep. That is if we do not allow the intuitive brain to give way to purely spiritual or religious matters, but ground ourselves in the material aspects of existence, some forms of recreation and entertainment which would otherwise have us give way to fanaticism and fits of ecstasy; nor overdevelop the intellectual brain with laborious studies and the mundane concerns of life.

Confused dreams are the result of an overwrought nervous system, brought on mainly by the day-time stresses of over activity upon the frontal brain and wrong cultivation, distorts the sensitive cerebellum while it sleeps. Subsequently, weakened through neglect which leads to its inactivity, the intuitive brain absorbs the strong radiation from the frontal brain simultaneously with the experience of the spirit, creating a mixture like a double exposure on a photographic plate.

This double influence is manifested in the frequent appearance in dreams of words and sentences; in that, words only originate in the activity of the frontal brain. Only the frontal brain forms words and sentences, because it is more closely bound to world of relativity.

The dangerous consequence of such an abnormal state for mankind, is that we are no longer susceptible to spiritual warnings and instructions through the intuitive brain in dreams. This inadequacy which endangers all humanity could otherwise be escaped through spiritual warning. Today only animals, which are animistic species, pick up this slack. They teach and warn us of impending dangers.

When, with the simplicity of a child, that is, with purity, we absorb everything fully and experience it immediately within ourselves, knowledge streams back through the intuitional brain to the intellectual brain. From there it serves as a strong and successful defense. This also increases our receptive capacity, depending on the nature of the outward happening. When the effects of our daily activities upon the day-brain produce great upbuilding effects for humanity as a whole, the stimulus of this day-consciousness reaches the cerebellum and enlightens our dreams.

Therefore, to create the ideal state of the nervous system, a state which will maintain that level of activity of intuitive perception of the spirit in the day-to-day experience is to balance intellect and spirit, manifested in clear and informative dreams. It is within our capacity – through our volition, our lifestyle and choice of foods – to govern the nervous system to a state that will permanently allow the level of intuitive perception to be maintained in the day-consciousness of thinking, and also of the dream state. We should not allow our nerves to become overwrought through the one-sided intellectual over cultivation, a condition which only gives rise to morbid imaginations we see, especially in art today.

Memory

With all the promotion of herbal remedies to increase microcirculation of the brain – yes, the herb ginkgo biloba has proven most effective in correcting circulatory disturbances (arterial and peripheral), arteriosclerosis, weakness in concentration *etc.*, – however, memory remains a fluid activity of the intuitive brain patterning. The back brain alone possesses the capacity to keep memories undistorted, a task impossible for the intellectual brain. The back brain alone is capable of retaining in pictures and intuitive perceptions of all happenings and experiences as such, and in such a manner that they can be exactly reproduced at any time as they really are, unchanged and undimmed.

The frontal brain cannot do this, because it is more closely bound to the gross material conceptions of time and space, *i.e.,* of relativity. It was not designed for reception, but for transmission of earthly things. Therefore, the key to a sharp memory is not to think too much. When we empty our minds of thoughts, intuitive perception will prompt us with that which is to be remembered. Sometimes questionable descriptions of what we say we experienced and heard are transmitted from a deficient memory. This is due to the impaired co-operation of the neglected intuitive brain, which consequently becomes degenerate and incapable of playing its full part. So we use opinions to supplement this deficiency, using words as clothing.

We find this deficiency in the words or writings of another based on their observation of what they believed they have seen or heard, no matter if it was only a moment past. The reproductions never accord with the original sense, it always introduces alterations. Even if only new words are used, the original meaning is entirely changed, sometimes distorted, although the speaker or writer may be absolutely willing to answer for it.

Allow weeks and months to elapse to read or hear of something. Even if it the experience happened, the explainer is unable to describe without error what was experienced or heard; one can never repeat it literally word for word. Much less if there are two, three, four or even ten persons who simultaneously heard or saw the same thing, they will give just as many different reasons for it.

This should serve to show why we cannot afford to get caught up in calculated thinking of the intellectual brain, but trust in the spontaneity of intuitive perception to bring about the right self-conscious action. Intuitive perception will surely find the right way if we ourselves do not wall it in. We must become free spirits, we must let the spirit have its way, especially in the case of deficient memory.

Refined Carbohydrates - Their Effect on Mental Health

Refined starches prevent the proper digestion and utilisation of protein, which subsequently depletes the body's supply of phosphorus in the body fluids; in that, the first step in the oxidation of glucose is formation of a phosphate ester which binds itself to calcium, transporting it to the bones, structural tissues and the nervous system. For calcium to be transported in the blood it has to bind itself to protein. X-rays have recently discovered small mineral particles – especially calcium is deposited in the pineal gland – explaining why as melatonin declines with advancing age, osteoporosis sets in due to the body's depletion of calcium. We can seethe correlation between refined sugars, not only to premature ageing, but to mental disorders as well – and are linked to the nature of our thoughts and perceptions that influence the hypothalamus to indulge in such foods.

The overindulgence in refined carbohydrates also causes a deficiency in essential nutrients, especially vitamin B, needed to stimulate the central nervous system, ultimately activating the brain. A deficiency of B vitamins impairs the metabolism of carbohydrates into glycogen by the liver. Most of the glucose obtained from glycogen conversion is used in the functioning of the nervous system, a deficiency which leads to its impairment.

Just as it is important for glucose to be available for the nervous system, so must the latter have the ability to utilise this nutrient. Where there is a deficiency of B vitamins, the utilisation of glucose by nervous tissue can decrease by 50 to 66%. One can therefore understand, not only the serious physiological effects of refined sugars on the development and maintenance of the brain and nervous system (beginning from infancy), but also the behavioral and neurological disquietude within those who have the poor availability in glucose and/or poor utilisation.

Classification of the Mental Bodily Temperament

Although the build of certain features of all higher organisms over the long chain of evolution is linked to the design and function of the nervous system, which in turn affect peculiarities of behavior, there are, however, some individuals, according to phrenology (see Appendix), whose body forms conform to more brain (nervous activity) over matter (than size). As Fowler explains, they:

> 7 Have a small stature; light built; small bones and muscles; a slim, tall, spare, sprightly person; quickness in motion; great physical activity; too much for strength; sharp features; thin lips; small, pointed nose; and sharp teeth, liable to premature decay. Are characterised mentally by a predominance of mind over body, so that its states affect the body more than the body does the mind; are in the highest degree susceptible to the influence of stimuli, and of all exciting causes; are, however, refined and delicate in feelings and expression, and easily disgusted with anything coarse, vulgar, or out of taste; enjoy and suffer in the highest degree; are subject to extremes of feeling; have the disgusts, sympathies, and prepossessions easily excited; experience a vividness and intensity of emotion, and a clearness, pointedness, and rapidity of thought, perception, and conception, and a love of mental exercise imparted by no other temperament; have a deep flow of pure and virtuous feeling, which will effectually resist, vicious inclinations; intense desires, and put forth correspondingly vigorous efforts to gratify them; are eager in pursuits, and feel that their ends are of the utmost importance, and must be answered now; are thus liable to overdo, and prematurely exhaust the physical powers, which are poor at best; are very fond of reading and study, of thinking and reasoning, of books and literary pursuits, of conversion, and of all kinds of information, and apt to lie awake at night, thinking, or feeling, or reading; inclined to some profession, or light mental occupation, such as administrative assistant, merchant, teacher, or if a mechanic, should be a goldsmith, or architect, or something requiring light action, but not

hard lifting, in other words, more head work than hand work; should, however, avoid close application; take much pleasurable recreation and exercise; practice deep breathing and find yourself as much as possible in high altitudes, mountain air, breezy climates and scenic surroundings; protect the vital parts of the body (brain, eyes, sex organs, breast) from washing with harmful substance, extreme temperatures, long exposure to the sun – though short and adequate sunshine helps metabolism; stop using the motor force of the brain as in leadership, driving in traffic, high pressured working environment, lecturing, gossiping, and the demanding responsibilities of executive positions; endeavor to enjoy existence; and avoid being worried; maintain that requisite balance between rest and activity; avoid all kinds of stimulants, wines, tobacco, tea and coffee included; with head as delicate as stomach, should basically stick to a bland diet.

6 Are like 7 in character, only less in degree; more given to intellectual and moral than animal pleasures, and action than rest; cannot endure slow or stupid employees; with the motive 6, are of good size; rather tall, slim, lean, and raw boned, if not homely and awkward; have prominent bones and features, particularly front teeth and nose; a firm, straightforward, rapid energetic walk; great ease and efficiency of action, with little fatigue; a keen penetrating eye; large joints, hands, feet, *etc.*, a long face and head, and high head and forehead; a brain developed more from nose over the occiput than around the ears; strong desires, and great power of will and energy of character; vigorous passions; a natural love of hard work, and capacity for carrying forward and managing great undertakings; that thorough-going spirit which takes right hold of great projects with both hands, and drives into and through thick and thin, in spite of obstacles and apposition, however great, and thus accomplishes wonders; superior business talents; unusual strength and vigour of intellect; strong common sense; good general judgement; with a cool, clear, long calculating head; a reflective, planning, discriminating cast of mind, and talents more solid than brilliant; are more fond of natural science than literature; of philosophy than history; of the deep, solid branches than the belles-lettres; of a professional and mental than laborious vocation; of mental than bodily action; and the moral than sensual.

5 Have a good, fair muscles; are quite prominent-featured, easy of motion, enduring, tough, hardy, clear-headed, and fond of intellectual pursuits; have good ideas, and excellent native sense and judgement; talk, speak, and write to the purpose, if at all; love action and exercise, and walk and work easily; are efficient, and capable of doing up a good life labor, but not of a genius. With the vital 6, are sprightly, lively, vivacious, and happy; and with the motive 3, are more adapted to a life of labor, but should chose some office business, yet exercise a great deal – no matter how much.

4 Have fair mental action, if circumstances fully call it forth; if not, are commonplace; must depend on talents more on culture and plodding studiousness than natural genius; with culture, can do well, without it little; with the motive and the vital 6 or 7, are far better adapted to farming or manual pursuits than literary, and should cultivate intellect and memory.

3 Have little love of literary pursuits; are rather dull, and fall asleep over books and sermons; and cannot marshal ideas for speaking or writing.

2 Are exceedingly dull of comprehension; slow of perception; poor in judgement and memory; hate books; must be told what and how to do; and should seek direction form superior minds.

1 Are almost senseless and idiotic.

The ultimate goal of the human-spirit, is to cultivate the intellect in such a way that there is established harmony among the rays of expressions – like notes of a melodious chorus. One will have attained Christ-consciousness.
In the words of Fowler,

> Is by far the best, that most favorable to true greatness and general genius, to strength of character, along with perfection, and harmony and consistency throughout, is one in which each is strongly marked, and all about equally developed.
>
> Excessive motive with deficient mental gives power with indolence, so that the talents lie dormant. Excessive vital gives physical power, and enjoyment, but too little of the mental and the moral, along with coarseness and animal passions. Excessive mental confers too much mind for body, too much intellectual aspirations, sentimentalism and exquisiteness, along with green house precocity. Whereas their equal balance gives an abundant supply of vital energy, physical stamina, and mental power and susceptibility. They may be compared to the several parts of a steamboat and its appurtenances. The vital is the steam-power; the motive, the hulk or frame-work; the mental, the freight and passengers. The vital predominant generates more animal energy than can be well worked off, which causes restlessness, excessive passion, and a pressure which endangers outbursts and overt actions; predominant motive gives too much frame and hulk; moves slowly, and with weak mental, is too light freighted to secure the great ends of life; predominant mental overloads, and endangers sinking; but all equally balanced and powerful, carry great loads rapidly and well, and accomplish wonders. Such persons unite cool judgement with intense and well governed feelings; great force of character and intellect with perfect consistency; scholarship with sound common sense; far-seeing sagacity with brilliancy; and have the highest order of both physiology and mentality. It is said that such a tem-

perament belonged to the immortal Washington, and his character corresponded.

Most diseases, too, are consequent on this predominance or deficiency of one or another of these temperament, and when either fail, all fail. Hence the infinite importance of cultivating those that are weak.

7 or 6 Are uniform, consistent, harmonious in character, even-tempered, popular, and generally liked; not remarkable for any specialities of talents of character, nor for any deficiencies, and "maintain the even tenor of their way" among men.

5 or 4 Are in the main consistent, and in harmony with themselves, but more or less affected by circumstances; show general uniformity of life and doctrine, but different circumstances change their characters.

3 Have uneven heads and characters; are singular in expression, looks, and doctrine, and variable in conduct; often inconsistent, and with excitability (intensity of feeling, as well as temper) 6 or 7, the creatures of circumstances; take one-sided views of things; are poor counselors; need and should take advice; are very warped in judgement; propound strange ideas, and run after novelties; and need to cultivate unity and homogeneity of opinion and conduct.

2 Are like three, only more so; are nondescripts; idiosyncratic in everything; just like themselves, but unlike anybody else; and neither like, nor are liked by, others.

TO CULTIVATE – Exercise the weaker and restrain the stronger faculties and temperament according to directions in this work.

PART THREE

THE SEVEN PLANES OF HUMAN DEVELOPMENT

Humans are a microcosm of their Universe. A world to themselves annexed through their basic species to other forms and genera; an origin of the *beau ideal* of human perfection. Part I looked at this perfection in form covered in four basic cloaks – the animistic, ethereal, astral and the physical. However, these cloaks are actually seven and form seven planes of human development.

The number seven symbolises this perfection: "And on the seventh day God ended His work which He had made" (Gen. 2:2). Seven becomes the governing number in all Creation. Wherever there is perfection, it indicates the Will of God working. In that the *original* human form, the ethereal, was created perfect, just as the Creator rendered it when He bestowed on us all the same gifts and talents, our present imperfections point to our departure from the Divine ordinance of things – *the ideal*. So for us to gain self-perfection, we must ascend seven flight of steps, by living according to the requisitions of perfection, which is as far as we live perfect lives.

In every strata of Creation lies this perfection, there are:

1. seven universes of the world described as churches – Ephasus (encompassing earth), Smyrna, Pergamos, Thyatira, Sardis, Philadelphia, Laodicea (Rev. 1:11).
2. seven major musical notes – do, re, me, fa, so, la, ti, do.
3. seven colours of the rainbow – red, orange, yellow, green, blue, indigo, violet.

4. seven day cycle called a week – Monday, Tuesday, Wednesday, Thursday, Friday, Saturday, Sunday.
5. seven endocrine glands – pineal, pituitary, thyroid, thymus, pancreas, gonads, adrenals – each concerned with radiating the blood.
6. seven energy centres (chakras) – crown, brow, throat, heart, solar plexus, sacral, base – meridian points of the astral body running vertically along the spinal column of the central nervous system, each connecting to its respective endocrine gland.
7. seven senses – hearing, touch, sight, taste, smell, clairvoyance, clairaudience.
8. seven parts of life-form – embryo, amniotic fluid, amnion, yolk sac, allantois, chrion, albumnious fluid.
9. seven human spirit planes – Paradise, Fine Ethereal Matter, Medium Ethereal Matter, Coarse Ethereal Matter, Fine Dense matter, Medium Matter, Coarse Dense matter.

Humans, the crown of Creation, have united in themselves all the species and all the worlds that lay in Creation. Our incarnation into flesh and blood links the Ethereal World of Matter (soul) with Coarse Dense Matter (body), while our roots remain in the higher Spiritual Plane (Paradise). Therefore, we can explore these worlds in our growth toward self-consciousness.

This is the beauty of being intuitive-perceptive beings. Not the materialists we have become, following our base passions and drives we sells our souls – as if to slavery – for the pleasures of the World of Dense Matter – the first, second and third planes – which has only served to weaken our spirit and cut us off almost entirely from our roots. Imprisoned and constrained we stagger under our heavy burden, groping about for whatever pleasure we can find, hoping to quench our spiritual barenness by accumulating material possessions, seeking fame and weakening comfort. We have become so greedy in our pleasure pursuits, we now find our spirit trapped and subjugated to the dying form of our animal passions, for they are the only pictures our thought conjures in periods of quiet comfort, which like a narcotic is hostile to the spirit , which paralyses our will for meaningful activity.

Thus Ethereal Matter, the fourth, fifth and sixth steps on the ladder to self-consciousness, came into being – intermediary steps with cherubim and the flaming sword to bar any ascent to the seventh, unless we transmute our base passions in the fire of volition. Painfully must we work our way up these fiery steps through a change in our desires and activities, to be purified like rare gold, to regain our spiritual heritage.

Through the seven planes of human development, it is possible to experience all these spheres due to the nature of our being – intuitive perception, thoughts and deeds. The substances of each of these planes form our cell molecular structure – DNA – all depending on our level of consciousness, *i.e.*, spiritual maturity. They form the blueprint of genetic disposition to the moral advancement of the soul. Within each of these seven planes are again seven minor steps to complete each stage of this progress.

The Seven Planes of Human Development

1. Spiritual Plane or Paradise (the highest plane of the human spirit-germ in unconscious origin, and to where we return as self-conscious beings in completing its cycle in Ephasus

(bridge of animistic substantiality connecting spirit to materiality)

2. Fine Ethereal Matter (source of bliss-consciousness, the ideal human being, the rapture)
3. Medium Ethereal Matter (source of transcendental consciousness, self-perfection)
4. Coarse Ethereal Matter (source of pure intuitive perception, love, wisdom, logic)
5. Fine Gross Matter (source of thought, feeling and temperament)
6. Medium Gross Matter (source of words, emotions, self-care)
7. Coarse Dense Matter (source of action, physicality, relativity)

THE FIRST PLANE - PRIMARY OR PRIMITIVE DEVELOPMENT

This is the grounding or primeval plane of human development which places man in direct contact with their surroundings and Nature. This takes into account social and family affections – parental love, love of children, the young and pets. The desire here is for friendships and associations, and a community of feeling and interest; love of country, home, where one lives and has lived – our adaptation to the need of an abiding place in which to exercise family feelings; polygamy; patriotism *etc.*, this plane represents healthy childhood, connoted also to primitive humans, our dependency and imitative instinct.

It is for this reason this first plane relates to the nerve meridan at the base of the spine, also called sacral *chakra* – the lower animal self. From here the spinal column leads to the brain to form the complete central nervous system, which then branches into the posterior parasympathetic nerve branch to bring sensations to the body; at the same time it connects us to our dormant higher spiritual self through the intuitive back brain, where it climaxes at the crown chakra and represents the seventh plane.

The natural connection to the higher self, creates the instinct that binds us to worship. So here you find individuals with childlike, simplistic blind faith, content to look like children for succor; be it to a religious sect, angels and deities, and the almost servile worship of God. Hence the primitive worship of gods, demi-gods, celestial beings, and ancestors. Just like children who are dependent upon parents for security and expect fairy-like magic in times of need and danger, so do men of simple faith seek the animistic *(of the gods and deities)*; the guidance of departed souls and deities *etc.*

This plane is spiritual development at its lowest. In fact, the spirit-seed with its protective astral animistic and ethereal bodies is yet to be awakened. Human nature is as coarse as gross matter itself, wanting in refinement and beauty.

This first plane represents childhood at its full development by age seven. However, there are seven other intermediary plane within this and the other planes of development, the development process which can take seven times seven times seven years – thus a cyclic age of a life-time for an individual, or centuries for particular races or nations. In such cases reference is made to the childish, backward or primitive.

The consciousness of a primitive people is no more advanced than that of a child. Such speaks to stagnation or spiritual retrogression. The first stages of development of all human life, which spanned millions of years, crowds into today's child who bears the experiences of former lives slumbering within the spirit awaiting an awakening.

Still, in most adults, their belief systems are built upon understandings gained only from this first human life-cycle. Conditionings to which one adheres without examining their authenticity, and by adulthood, they still hold such to as personal conviction. Not only individuals become stuck in their development for their entire life-cycle, collective races or homogenous groups of people experience no growth of the intellect, feelings and emotions, no spiritual awakening and in the law of development, and must eventually face extinction.

To understand development on this plane, study the development of a child, whose thinking does not greatly differ from the highly developed animal. For this reason the child has little responsibility towards the Laws of Creation (from which human laws devolve) which demands taking responsibility for actions.

A child only affects its environment through its[23] animistic or elemental faculties. In healthy surroundings it roams as animals do; talks to flowers and butterflies; enjoys rolling in the mud or getting soaked in the rain – establishing that firm connection with Nature – which is fundament of primeval life. But children can be just as cunning as animals which leads to dishonesty in adult life if there is no further development in consciousness. It is said: innocence bears cruelty within.

The beauty of a healthy, natural development shows itself only at puberty when selfish development begins. Animistic activity affects the forming of thought-patterns, which shapes one's reality.

If this natural development is arrested, we get an adolescent's perception of reality that is out of order, out of control – the id or childish quality that "enjoys smashing toys." Then comes the abusive, oppressive and anti-social behavioral patterns – total disregard for the feelings of others, animals or the environment. All because they did not have the right childhood foundation on which to truly experience real life. These are the children who grow up to become narcissists, head totalitarian regimes and commit all kinds of atrocities against humanity.

But it also happens that no matter how correctly guarded and nurtured is one's childhood development, a child could turn out to be the "black sheep" of the family. This is due to the attraction of a child with an inferior mind. A soul born with the hidden propensity to kill, steal and wreak within the home and society. Although this plane is the foundation for individuality and the idiosyncrasies of the soul, the true nature of the latter does not break through the intuitive perceptions until the juvenile stage of an individual or race. One is, at this stage, incapable of refined self-conscious actions, so they live what they learn, which, too often, are the propensities of the brute.

This is why it is critical to govern children by moral suasion *vs.* rod, patience *vs.* scolding, directing vs. crushing will in the formative period cycle. We must encourage right actions by rewards instead of wrong ones by punishment. In addition, we must choose for them the right nourishment and outdoor activity for the proper forming of physical features and securing of a strong mind. And, children must also be allowed to be children and not prematurely dragged up into a grownup world.

It was the same guidance extended to primeval humans who in their childlike faith were connected to and worshipped the gods and goddesses in a healthy and unrestrained way. Accordingly they were able to absorb the animistic rays to develop their mental faculties. The result was knowledge in horticulture, farming, pottery, jewellery making, fine fabrics, *etc.*, even superior to some of the works of art of today.

However, history records how missionaries assisted governments in implementing assimilationist policies and practices, forcibly removed children of many races and tribes from their homes and placed into government and religious institutions. The underlying position was that conversion to Christianity required the weakening of the spiritual influence of the elders and culture, which they deemed primitive, on the younger generation. They saw the physical separation of the younger children from their family as necessary for spiritual development. Over time, some began to believe the erroneous views about their own racial inferiority and supported those missions.

Regardless of how noble was their intention, if such was ever the case, these missionaries violated the Laws of Creation with their approach. For this reason they could not then, nor can they today, achieve living results. Empty queues on Sundays speak for themselves. The missionaries, lack of knowledge, *i.e.*, of the *gods* and *deities* or *celestial archetypes* of peoples, show up those so-called primitive people, who then and today still stand in the archaic knowledge, to be more valuable in Creation than one who merely adhered to the acquired Christian faith, disregarding that which is animistic and treating such as myths and fairy-tales.

This smooth transition in the growth of consciousness, after hundreds of years, still must to be applied today if there is be any progress for those so affected. For in the law of development, where there exists any gap, where any rung from the ladder to progress is removed, only failure ensues in further development. What remains is flimsy support, which gives way as one attempts to climb.

Progress can only happen gradually, particularly when it involves uplifting and furthering races and peoples who have lagged behind in their spiritual development or who, because of their spiritual indolence, have retrogressed and are incarnated once more to a lower stage. Real building can only begin at that stage which has already been fully experienced and grasped.Omitting any stage obstructs all progress. Centuries of slavery, colonization and occupation now bear witness to those uprooted from tradition or those who conform to alien doctrines and teachings, that they have only become imitators or submissive in spirit; denying themselves of the possibility to mature to self-consciousness.

To conform, especially to alien doctrines and lifestyles, is to become submissive in spirit, and deny oneself the possibility to mature to self-consciousness. To resign oneself to live from any other place other than that which allows for the right to self-determination, is like selling oneself into slavery. It is self-delusion or hypocrisy, and many today live this lie. One merely imitates. Such life breeds a false sense of self - the lack of ambition. For behind all submissive resignation resides distrust, cunning, lust, conceit or malice.

To live under submission is not living from a "spiritual" place, our true existence. There can be no loyalty in the spirit, as is observed in the false sense of self - the lack of race pride of many, or wanting to remain indigenous or embracing traditional values. To be somebody usually involves becoming like their mentor, oppressor (former or current), to look like them, to dress like them, to own what they own, to strive for the same ideals, for they symbolise the ideal human.

Hence the tendency to conform, to imitate – the one trait underdeveloped human and animal share. Even at a biological adult age most adults are very *childish*; submerged in the social situations that continuously influence and shape their identity. An existence void of free will to affect meaningful action to transform society for the self, to participate in social situations and deal with them critically.

Nothing is wrong with the imitative instinct. It has its place on this primary plane of human development. This instinct has to do with human requisition for doing, talking, acting, *etc*.

Imitation forms the basis of self-control. It chastens the animal faculties to bring out the natural talents and abilities, patterning, obtaining and acquiring whatever is beautiful and perfect, especially in the art, as in mimicking. It allows us to relate anecdotes to life with theatrical taste and talent. However, when perverted, it not only copies faults, but alien habits, customs, foreign fashion and architecture under the illusion of progress. So rather than refreshing difference indigenous to the various races and culture, we have uniformity, conformity.

Through Natural Laws, *every* creature is endowed with this *imitative instinct*, but only in the childhood cycle, to take the place of free will before it becomes active at the onset of puberty. Childhood is fundamental to this receptive capacity which youth is made of, which should be transmuted into self-conscious activities by the cycle of adulthood. The imitative instinct is the preparatory step in our inner development until the time when, in the case of animals, it is enriched and supported by experience, and in the case of humans, the greatest personal achievements.

The imitative instinct in human is today evident in the perfecting, not only of the human body, but also of our languages. The spirit forms the physical body, the noble form it has attained, in which the possibility exists to become even more beautiful. After *primeval spiritual-man and woman* received the animal bodies as earthly covering, in addition to the transformation of the animal-blood into human blood, they also brought about the development of language.

Bent at first like the animals, imitating sounds in Nature around them to express intuitive perception, wishes and thinking, to establish a common background of understanding, eventually the vocal organs formed along with the gradual upright human posture and the sinking of the larynx. The gradual sinking of the larynx brought about the difference in the outer form of the body of human and animal; for in animals, especially apes, there is no change in the position of the larynx. As the human larynx sank, the mouth was shaped, transforming the initial hoarse, epiglottal sounds into the complete voice and vowel ranges characteristic of humans alone.

Today this cycle is repeated in only a few short years beginning with the entry into earth-life of every first cry of a new born baby. Through imitation it learns to speak, passing through all the stages of development which took primeval humans millions of years.

From the end of the first year, up to about the eight or ninth, the larynx sinks in every child. A space forms at the back of the throat which allows for the free refined movement of the tongue, a space which is particularly important for the formation of different vowels. Apes, the closest animal to developed humans, do not have the vocal organ because they do not experience the descent of the larynx. Their epiglottis reaches right up to the palate, as with the vast majority of mammals, as they lack spirit to foster logical development.

Upon completing this plane of development of childhood, the nerve sheath of the spinal column serves as the channel through which generative power, also known as *kundalini* energy or serpent fire, flows. This signals the next progressive development from this primitive cycle of all individuals and races. Hence the gradual uncoiling of the serpent with the exercising of *free will*.

A hardy nervous system supports one's spiritual ascent up ladder in the quest for knowledge, for exploration of one's sexuality, for adventure and gradually opens the connection to the higher spiritual self where man closes this cycle as in a circle. A circuit of energy forms wherein the serpent's head (the intellectual masculine) surrenders or consummates with its own tail (the intuitive feminine) – the ultimate climax in the sphere of spiritual activity.

SECOND PLANE - THE EMOTIONAL/SELFISH (SELF-CARING) DEVELOPMENT

In the animal kingdom, by the time an offspring closes its dependent cycle it is impelled to mature on its own. It leaves its habitat or is expelled to begin to face its own experiences, to learn how to survive and grow strong. This is the law of development. No longer a child, the adolescent is, or should be, left to exercise free will. To prepare for this age of responsibility, the period of secondary education, or cultural juvenile initiations, mark the beginning of this young manhood and womanhood cycle, which peaks around the age of fourteen. This is the age for the development of ambition, dignity, and firmness, economy, commerce, fortunes, self-defense, *etc.*

Secondary education should cultivate self-control. Through observation and experience, youths gain basic knowledge of their unique nature. Education should guide youths how to carefully develop their capacity to observe themselves as well as their self-caring propensities.

But such training usually happens only in so-called archaic societies and cultures and not in today's modern culture. An era which sees children at the age of five or so instructed in sex education as part of curriculum, not to mention the psychic pollution coming out of Hollywood. Systems of education designed to create young adults with the precocity of hot-house plants. Though made to appear brilliant and wise, before long they usually learn how ill-prepared they really are on the inside to resist the dark influences around them, reaching out to them to pull them down. And it does not take much effort to bring about their destruction, for they have no firm root system, for they dis not gradually develop under exposure to wind and rain, much less storms.

Gone are the golden days of healthy logical development, of innocent awakening and intimate moments of self discovery. But the symbolic customs of initiation – however primitive – if omitted, is bound to engender emotional problems sooner than later whether in relationship to one's self or to others, as we so gravely observe in today's youth delinquency and anti-social behavior. For this plane concerns the awakening of sexuality and gender issues –

young manhood and womanhood. Human life must now adapt to Nature's male-female, sexual blending, affiliating, and creative ordinances. Concern for parental love shifts to that which attracts the opposite sex, and is attracted to it, admires and awakens admiration, creates and endows offspring, desires to love, be loved, and marry. It involves the conjugal instinct and talent, gallantry, womanliness, ladyism, maleness, gentlemanliness, passion.

Although this is the first etherised plane of human existence, in that it mirrors the soul, it remains part of Gross Matter, our animality. Thus called the plane of emotions – the astral plane of light. And just as we cannot see atomic energy but can perceive its effects, so is it for the effects of light refraction of the soul, giving rise to our astral light-energy.

Hence the inexplicable charm of unadulterated youths. The warmth and vitality that radiates in their personality. Some call it personal magnetism, the flowering of sexuality, the awakening to self-conscious action. Generative power is the catalyst to this self-consciousness. The awareness of our perception of reality in our everyday experiencing. The nature of this conscious awakening provides the magnet of our sexuality, that is, makes us attractive or repulsive. The biological changes are but the after-effects of light radiations, the development of procreative organs and faculties for the preservation of our creations.

As already stated sexuality, however, does not speak to sexual instinct which ensures this procreative act, or what is termed "sexy". It is not about femaleness or maleness, nor one's sexual proclivity. But speaks to *the nature of one's activity in which we choose to engage based on gender.*

In other words, in becoming self-conscious of gender, mainly in which direction we strive to develop the abilities – in the compelling and energetic masculine (positive) or the quiet, preserving feminine (negative) way – the spiritual life. The urge for sexual intercourse could therefore be called material or nature, and should remain where it belongs – secondary to the creative endeavors.

Self-conscious actions are what we entered this life to perform, if we are to be considered human beings and not animals. Only through the nature of our activity does our spirit form us into human beings, conscious of our personality. From the point of human origin, the development of the desire of our primordial spirit-seed, arose from its urge to ego-consciousness in the pursuit of knowledge in the World of Matter. This achievement is the only standard of value whereby one is considered a person. It is based *on the quality of the activity* in which one is engaged. And sexuality alone determines this value. It literally controls our entire being.

Sexuality embodies those means employed by the Creator of all life for its inception – for the perpetuity and multiplication of all forms of life. It creates in each sex admiration and love for the other; renders woman receptive, winning, persuasive, urbane, affectionate, loving, and lovely; develops feminine charms and graces; wields supreme control over the voice, walk, dance, beauty, complexion, eyes. It makes man noble in feeling and bearing; elevated in inspiration; gallant, tender, and bland in manner, courageous; affectionate toward woman; highly susceptible to female charms and friendliness; and clothes him in dignity, power, and persuasiveness.

Overall gender wields supreme control over talents, temperament, perceptions, morals, happiness and every element of body and mind. Factors which form, or should form, the basis for sexual attraction.

The desire for sexual union, however, gives us the freedom to unite in various ways, which brings about different realities. Hence, there is no right sexual state, and the wrong one can only self-destruct. To claim the rightness of a sexual state is to live one-sidedly in some compressed definition which merely serves a social order and counters the Laws of Nature. For, based on the *nature* of ability and distinct characters, there is not only one compliment existing for any individual, but many, so that a person seeking a compliment is not merely limited to one particular person. Many opportunities arise in our lifetime and unite in various ways, bringing about different realities, different sexual states, with each choice we make.

For hybrids, that is, individuals who are part male and part female in the mind-body relationship, their gender attraction is of a different kind. It is attraction with a distortion at the soul level, which also shows in an abnormal development of the brain.

In the case of the woman, it results from her striving to show or push male characteristics to the foreground and vice-versa for the male. These individuals find it increasingly difficult to establishing meaningful, healthy relationships. In fact, they are repulsed by those of the opposite sex who are genuinely male or female. Any union with another of the opposite sex usually bears the same distortion at the soul level. A strong woman attracted to a weak man or a homosexual union.

Since sexual union should come after a spiritual union, that is, the result of an attraction of the complimentary qualities of the soul to bring about oneness and completeness through the exchange of energy, this kind of attraction is therefore unnatural. Sexual unions that do not stem from the *desire for union* of the split parts of a definite species of full value are mainly a sexual propensity, a need with an "ego" to feed.

Then again one would argue that only opposite poles can attract; whereas like ones repel. But only if the sexual attraction is from the level of what meets the eye and not that both (in the case of homosexual union – one) bear a distortion at soul level. Male and female are split species. It is why all human cells (except sex cells) contain 46 chromosomes. Sperm cells and egg cells in humans have only 23 chromosomes each. This makes complete what is but split species each – male and female. If a sexual union is not for striving again for the formation of a complete species[24], for the liberation of the souls concerned, its purpose is basically for physical pleasure or some material benefit. Hence the so-called love lives, destined to gloom, anguish, sorrow and ever greater longing; for they are not complimentary unions, wherein both work together to achieve something perfect.

Though sexual attraction confers procreative capacity and conjugal talents, it also engenders platonic love. A union wherein two not only joyfully and voluntarily serve each other, but grow together towards spiritual ennoblement. They surrender personal desires and as it is said: "wait hand and foot on the other".

For this reason the hypothalamus gland is located at the lowest section of the brain, the seat of physical life and apex of every mental organ. For while this animal and its social organ is to man what foundations are to houses – absolutely indispensable – yet it, and others like it, bears a higher quality to human moral faculties than to our animal ones, to those that ally us more to animistic beings, angels, and God than to the temporal, to spirituality than to sensuality, and therefore is the common sentient of mankind.

A healthy development on the first plane, through which one has enjoyed closeness to Nature, family and a stable home, determines how we face reality at this critical turning point. It fosters understanding of the right kind of paring in Nature and the home. It allows for the spirit to come consciously and positively to life.

The impulse to meaningful life is therefore based on the experiences of our formative years, experiences which should have been completed by the beginning of this stage to self-consciousness. If one is brought up badly or is misguided, he or she lacks that solid foundation or upbringing of communal sharing and healthy relationships. Childhood experiences should form a solid bridge to develop the intuitive capacity for real experiencing. Without this, the foundation needed for meaningful contribution to societal life is shaky or missing and the spiritual will power to govern bodily urges and desires is weak or absent.

What should become a pure innocent awakening toward spiritual self-consciousness turns into animal-like passions for life, instincts that pull and tug at our soul until it corrupts our magnetism. For along with sexual instinct, the selfish propensities create and awaken our animal desires and instincts, and we supply for those wants, especially for our physical necessities. Pudency which arises with sexual instinct gives way to debauchery. The inability to forge meaningful relationships results in quarrels, malice, divorce, *etc;* oppressive acts of rape, sabotage, slander, war – religious, ideological, even scientific. An adolescent's corrupt desires and passions can be allowed to increase in such a way that even the young man or woman is seized with self-horror.

Such youths find it difficult to act responsibly. The decision to do wrong shows that the individual is either gravely evil or has no will, low moral development. For responsibility begins with each resolution we make in life, not just from the consequences of the resolution. Will power drives resolution to become an accomplished deed. Those who act irresponsibly shows that their wrong desires influence their free will instead of the other way around, and in such a way that it takes a predictable direction, just like animals. Their free will becomes so oppressed that they cannot act in a creative and progressive way.

This is what leads many to say life is unfair, there is no free will or we do not have choices, we are mere "pawns in the hand of fate". So we readily submerge our already weak, defective character and conform to the influences of our surroundings.

It is our emotions that render our constitution weak or strong. Because the emotions reflect the nature of the soul on this plane, dark emotions cloud our already weak perceptions, giving way to all kinds of error and unsound judgement. The Darkness seeks to lay claim to such a soul, even if the individual does not want evil.

If one does not want good, the spirit struggles within to be free of this paralysing Darkness. In this confused state, many can no longer listen to the quiet inner voice which speaks to them, so as to establish a spiritual connection or develop trust in a higher guidance. Many lean on their own understanding or, if they do believe in some form of guidance, they only seek endorsement and support for their wrong choices and rush into danger with their eyes bandaged by lust, pride and ignorance.

This only leads to that stage where they can no longer do the right thing. In survival consciousness they over-develop the combative and destructive propensities given to them for self-defense and keen thinking, in a negative way. Until, of course, there comes a mental breakdown. The brain, designed as the steering element to spiritual understanding –and releases "mental anarchy" upon the psyche – the soul's perception – and paralyses it. Within this paralysis lies the killer narcissistic, oppressive, warlike, cruel, compulsive, deceptive, distrustful individual – a danger to themselves and others even if they could avoid many things with a little self-education and show consideration for others.

Such behavior plunges any individual, homogenous group or nation back into the Dark Ages, when oppression and cruelty and greed spread their dark wings over humanity – even more so than today. In this depraved condition, marked by the inability to do the right thing, one no longer desires to continue living and seeks suicide as a way out. Not before, however, in cases of totalitarian regimes, they plunge entire nations into poverty, suffering and misery.

Regardless of how low is a genetic breeding or how poor the childhood upbringing, with the right education or psycho-analysis at this critical point, designed so that the higher virtues are allowed to reach the soul, the overculivated destructive selfish propensities can be restrained to the point where they are aligned with the nobler intuitive perceptions of the soul. With continuous striving the forces of good and evil will be equally balanced within the being and free will again established.

With the perpetual desire to do good, any individual will be able to conquer evil propensities inherent in the World of Matter. No longer susceptible to corrupt personal magnetism, one attracts luminous rays of help and higher intelligence from on high. Celestial, animistic and human beings bearing the help and guidance we seek, all based on the particular emotions of the soul. We can gain the victory of good over evil at anytime, but only if we strive to do the right thing.

Life then earns new value through this striving upwards, and a delightful, vital warmth pulsates through all earthly joys and pleasures. Hence an ardent love of life, often ending in jubilant enthusiasm for all that exists and is proffered.

THIRD PLANE - THE INTELLECTUAL OR MENTAL PLANE

Development on this plane endows sagacity upon the intellect, the keen execution of the fertile masculine principle of thought extension and structural organisation. Here develops the ability to use Divine precepts to classify and organise thought into a matrix of energy beneficial to any required design. This third plane is the sphere of action that drives or influences the second – the emotional plane. If we call the former plane the gate of the soul, then this intellectual plane is the actual gateway, the passage of knowing where deep levels of spiritual understanding may be brought forth, where perceptions are expanded and utilised as head and heart become one.

Energetically, it's path leads from the solar plexus (the gut) via nerve impulses and connects to the conscious brain, through the higher, intuitive perceptive brain. The nature of the relationship between the two brains determines the quality of mentality. It's highest boundary, that is, where mind ends, soul begins – the midpoint of development of the same personality, the well balanced mind being one in which both states (intellect and intuition) are equally proportioned. On this plane feeling connects with the moral nature of things on higher planes, to be governed accordingly.

Because this is the plane of action, it is here the female who over-cultivates this masculine aspect of self represses her femininity. Through the perpetual motion of masculine things that occupies her thoughts, the cold, calculating intellect becomes over-developed to the point where it hardens and walls in her *delicate perceptions*.

And since physical forms go hand in hand with the development of spiritual self-consciousness in the body, this disposition does not bring about an immediate outward change in her feminine form, but subjects her spirit to this immediate change. The reason is, the dense material body is inert and therefore subject to very limited change. However, those born genetically predisposed to such *masculine* characteristics, although their physical body is markedly female, they tend to bear narrow hips and muscle tone like the male, as opposed to those women just beginning to strive in this direction.

The exception must be made, however, with those genuine women bearing the above features, resulting from over-breeding, also one-sided sports or wrong physical activities engaged in by their mothers. Here the consequences of the mothers "sins" are transferred to the children.

The woman who bears such a distortion of the soul is not strong in any direction as regards her thoughts and actions. Neither is she strong towards the male or female direction and this dichotomy remains her most bitter inner conflict. For it is a direction contrary to the initial desire of her primordial spirit-seed, which determined the sex she became in the World of Matter.

For no other reason does the intellect exist but for the development of the mind, the cultivation and restraint of temperament and feeling. It is that balance between coarser and finer, lower planes of our animality and the higher moral planes, it is the vehicle between the relative and the abstract, the conscious and the subconscious (perceptive). Its development opens the doors for all possibilities and demands a unity with Spirit in all thought and consequently all manifestation. A development which brings forth an understanding of the Natural Laws manifested through the masculine energy, and which requires crisp, clear and disciplined thought perception to utilise it to the fullest.

Though spiritualised, this plane is not and cannot become spiritual, even though it is the finest of material substance. For spirit and matter remain two different species which in the Law of Homogenous Species cannot mix, but together can produce new form. Take human temperament for example. They come about as a result of the intercourse between the unconscious etherised refraction of the soul (though the coarsest form) and the conscious material radiations of thought-flow patterns, which radiates the blood.

The faculty of intuitive perception on the next plane bridges these two existences – spirit and matter. It is the only faculty through which we can see ourselves for what we really are. It is akin to sightseeing unknown terrain where our mental acuity allows for each psychic experience, a brief look at the soul through the feelings of the body. A mental observation, however, can only teach us the thought meaning of things, not the emotional impression. The intellect can only tell us what we think about the scenery but not why it engenders particular feelings and emotions. And again, why the same experiences would evoke different emotions within another person viewing the same scene.

Normally the specific nature of the intellectual brain is to receive impressions from the intuitive brain, hold on to them, remodel them, and condense them according to the intellectual capacity to absorb. The intellectual brain can retain the experience as thought or transmit it through still further consolidation to be spoken or written word or direct action. It is an active process which the intellect itself does not understand.

An understanding comes only from the impression made, that is, pictures imprinted upon the soul – either spontaneously or after further reflection. These pictures emerge from the spirit which the brain uses to form conceptions. Therefore to be knowledgeable and wise, rests upon the observer's ability to analyse his or her personal experience. What or how a person experiences depends upon one's level of spiritual maturity.

Spiritual maturity concerns one's understanding of the masculine relation to the feminine creative principle of self. To understand the nature of unconscious spiritual things, one needs to recognise the limitations of the intellect. Being of a coarser and denser species it is only capable of perceiving relative comprehension of that which is material and not the underlying feminine creative principle, the wholly natural ordinance.

To strive to exercise intellectual dominance rather than establish equanimity of mind, comprehension happens only within the narrow confines of the dense material brain, and not the extended knowledge of its entire existence. Over time, an overgrowth of the conscious mind chokes off the intuitive bridge. What remains? A coarse, rough individual, deprived of any tenderness.

With the intellect acting as the driver instead of the steering mechanism of the vehicle transporting spirit, the occupant can only travel in the reverse, its most dependable course. For already, this is the role of the intellect, absorbing impressions or influences from the outside world to arrive at its own understanding.

To gain the correct understanding (always based on one's level of maturity to assimilate the impression received), the external occurance is sent to the intuitive brain, that is, reflected at the soul level to grasp its meaning. The interpretation then comes back as that cosy feeling, a sense that it feels right. However, this does not for a moment mean that the individual sees things the way they actually are, for knowledge is different on different levels of consciousness, but a least the observer can say "I experienced it". In other words, I experienced the unification and condensation of thought-concepts within me, I approached its realisation, hence created my reality, *condensed through my power*, what was in the beginning mere impression.

As the designated driver, the intellect places itself as a god upon pedestal, above the spirit – the reverse role. Here the observer tries to dissect and analyse things for themselves based only on their sagacity and does not pass it on to the spirit in its full value. Such understanding can only be distorted and the observer never comes to the point of experiencing. Their intellect serves no purpose but to inflate their ego. Instead of remaining unassuming, they glory in intellectual conceit about their own abilities. Without intercourse with the spiritual, their own power cannot rise, it merely reverses to exacerbate the emotional plane and chains them to their lust.

Hence, with thought-power we produce powerful forms to build our kingdom, *i.e.*, our circumstances, of good or evil. Like a photographic plate, our desires and wishes are taken over in pictures by the intellectual brain, exactly according to the volition that has issued from the emotions of the spirit. It then forms that pattern to be transformed or designed exactly corresponding to the thread of will, whether it becomes the spoken or written words or the impetus to action.

Hence planes one, two and three are not only closely connected and their effects interwoven, but also have more incisive and decisive effects on our lives than we could ever imagine. At this third level of consciousness are found the self-acclaimed advanced nations or people, stuck in their spiritual growth. The national thoughts are stimulated by the collective, base selfish desires and passions of the emotional plane. We only have to look at works of arts, fashion, literature, music, poetry, film and books. See how much thought-power is generated around nothing but sex, luxury foods and alcoholic beverages, creating abnormal desires from such artificial stimulation upon mind and body – to enfeeble the latter and overwhelm the nerves. It is that upon which we perpetually focus our thoughts and attract the conditions we experience in life.

For this reason, this plane of thought is where any attempt to bring about a body alignment must begin, in the exercising of self-control. The level of consciousness through which we may, through our thoughts, purify our dark emotions and lower animal passions. Sex has become such an obsession only because we think too much of it. If we again become ever watchful about what perpetually engages our thinking we can transmute lower dark energies – through the "twilight zone" – to higher spheres of light, of love, wisdom, logic, creativity.

It is all about exercising self-control. This is what living a *spiritual life* is about. If we strive to direct the lower energies upward, to be purified by the higher faculties of the soul such would give tremendous force of character and energy of the mind. Apart from being the serpent challenging our emotions to eat of the fruits of our base passions and desires, the intellect becomes the supreme warrior and destroyer of all that does not physically manifest for the good of the whole.

In guarding our thoughts, that is, being ever watchful of what emanates from our thinking, we can eradicate bad weeds before they take root in our consciousness as patterns which project themselves on the astral plane and are perceived by others around us in our aura or electromagnetic field in a repulsive manner. From this plane we can shed the egotistic desires in the aspiration of goodness for all; the virtues, purity, and moral principles. Until slowly, all thoughts, habits and aims for which we strive are transmuted by the higher mind, its counterpart.

Where the intellect dominates the intuitive brain, or vice-versa, to a grater degree, there is narrow-mindedness in one direction or the other and one is unable to be logical. When the intellect dominates, the individual becomes an intellectual, submitting in every respect to the capacity of the brain, confirming the ability to comprehend within the limited ability of the intellectual faculties. Though we may conscientiously seek truth, if the intellectual faculties are not aligned with the higher moral faculties, we experience only emotional blocks, errors. For no ray of truth can reach the soul and penetrate it, and everything we manifest is distorted and prejudiced. As the doorway of the soul, the imperfections of the intellect lock the soul in mental darkness, no matter how earnest the desire for light.

Therefore, maturity on this intellectual plane has nothing to do with scholastic abilities or associations with purely technological inventions. The ability called for here is to learn to refine the intuitive faculty to soar beyond the limits of comprehension, beyond time and space.

Emotions generated in times of terrible grief, major upheavals, severe suffering or supreme exhilaration can only help us transcend the dark layers of base feeling generated by thoughts, to give a glimpse of the condition of the soul. These are the invaluable opportunities which bring us in touch with our innermost self and leave us with intense longing for greater fulfilment in life.

If such moments are used to capture the conscious experience of a given time, we fortify the spirit and preserve its mobility for constant wakefulness towards ego-consciousness. Such an absorption not only serve as our strong and successful defense, it increases the receptive capacity of the mind. This is what makes the spirit *personal.* It gives it an individuality of its own. By so doing, we become more aware of our responsibility behind our intuitive perceptions, thoughts and actions; for with this kind of "seeing" comes with the possibility of developing our own personality for the strengthening of an independent capacity of decision-making.

In the forming of decision arising out of intense longing, we find the key to open the spiritual channels on which greater power can be mediated for all victory. First, the victory over the self, the carnal passions and lust, which will quickly awaken the spirit wanting to soar to new heights, so as to break the barriers of our self-imposed mental limitations. Only then can our spirit develop its full power and become what it should be. It is from this intercourse of mind we know that the spirit and the body are not one.

We cannot simply skip over the development of the intellect in striving to subjugate its radiations to that of our higher nature with simplistic faith. This can only lead to the fanaticism of the enthusiasts. Faith must be based upon a knowledge of the fundamental principles transformed into deed, *living* faith that permeates everything – all intuitions, all thoughts, all actions. The young woman and man strive only to develop those gifts and abilities which enable them to fulfil their *life's work and purpose.*

Only within a well governed intellect lies this power to execute the high art of judgment for our psychic defense and keen thinking, which surges to achieve our highest good. It gives correct judgement of the material properties of things and brings us in direct intercourse with the physical world; takes cognisance of the physical qualities of material things; and gives us an originating and practical cast of mind – the philosophising, penetrating, investigating kind.

Within the compass of the conscious mind are enormous expanses, intuitively immeasurable, in which we can sojourn and work, world without end. However, we cannot go beyond its capabilities intellectually, for beyond deals with the furthest recesses of the mind. To access and extend it further one must move in love at a level of complete surrender to intuitive perception of the next plane. Otherwise, we will remain caught between the boundaries of thought and emotions, each plane carrying their own limitations governed by our willingness or non-willingness to advance further.

In the logical course of things, this age of apprenticeship which cultivates the intellect whereby one's character is recognisable by the way they think, should have reached its peak by age twenty-one. But again, only if one wants to move away from the primitive planes of survival-consciousness, where mundane concerns and passions perpetually engross and influence the mind.

Still, it is better to properly develop oneself on the first two planes and only long for our further completion, than to develop the third plane and not align it with the fourth. The former planes, although called primitive and common-place by the intellectual, still hold full possibility for developing the strong, undimmed longing for self-conscious recognition. With good volition, this produces the cognition that leads to spiritual recognition at any moment, even within a few days, because the aspirants did not lose the firm ground under them.

The intellectuals on the other hand, though esteemed in the eyes of society, allows a narrowing of perception and therefore follows many a dangerous path on which their spirit is never able to unfold. When they recognise their error, their way back to the starting point becomes a maze from which attempts to escape lead only to sheer exhaustion. No energy remains to embark upon the real journey, for the soul no longer has its former vigour, and if it is not old age, it is stress-related illness and disease that set in as the body consumes itself prematurely.

To avoid overdevelopment, the intellect must equally developed with the next moral plane. Otherwise our selfish emotions influence our surroundings like a magnetic force that draws to ourselves all that is spiritually similar. It is this pull that is felt by others around us in our magnetic field; for each thought takes on form and strengthens itself on the emotional plane. It is called personal magnetism. We are either attractive or repulsive. Pleasant or unpleasant.

And what is drawn to us spiritually, eventually materializes in our lives, because a thought, sent out into different the "communities of thoughts", stays connected to us, the origin, radiating back through this link. Based on the nature of the emotions on the second plane of development, if we sow good or evil thoughts, in the Law of Returns, we reap the same conditions. Not, however, without influencing our surroundings, near or far, wherever others of like mind exist in this world.

Hence the allegory of the Tower of Babel which speaks to the human phylogeny, the "fall of man". It is about how material, sensually driven humans corrupt their magnetism and punish themselves. How they brought all kinds of travail to bear upon the soul by walking away from the childlike path of virtue of pure intuitive perception, thus shutting themselves out of Paradise from whence they descended in the quest for knowledge.

This is a story of man and woman coming to self-conscious. However, the woman, conscious of her sexual charm upon the man, calculated how she could exploit him sexually, and thus sold herself into coquetry. The man, in return sought to buy her for any price to be his possession (in some cultures as much as he can afford). With his spirit supplanted by the activity of the brain his sole desire became that of making himself sexually desirable through accumulating treasures and appropriating things of value – the picking and eating of "the apple" (Gen. 3:16).

No longer unassuming, his intellectual conceit about his own abilities and his own power took the place of that childlike simplicity, of faith and trust. Self-consciousness was no longer about selfless activity in the service of humanity, but to discover "himself" in his own activity, in his success, in everything he had achieved – everything went to his head, no longer acted from the heart.

With this humans began to build the tower of pride, greed and lust for power up to heaven, which had to be stopped. Hence the construction of what is called the City of Babylon. Suddenly people began to speak new languages: of greed, avarice, falsehood, jealousy, conceit, envy, robbery, hatred, arrogance, which brought other evil in its wake. No one understood the other anymore, nor did anyone take the pain to see about another's welfare. With the gift of *free will* given to humans as the determining factor for the path they choose to lead, their lives became their curse.

For this reason the fourth, fifth and sixth planes of the so-called beyond or heaven, emerged to ensure material humans never enter the Kingdom of Heaven without a change in attitude. Hence the words of Jesus: It is easier for a camel to enter through an eye of a needle than a materialist to enter the Kingdom of Heaven.

Choosing the sensual, materialistic path, compounded by poor upbringing and lack of childhood nurturing, creates a greater void, yearning to be filled. The self-caring instincts can only foster desires for personal fulfilment only – survival consciousness. Egocentricity takes the place of the self-culture; imagination replaces intuitive perception; splendor, vanity and extravagance replace the true sense of beauty. Satisfying the ego replaces the perpetual striving upward through loving, contributing activities in the service of genuine humanity. A striving which at the same time would raise the barrier of our strong will-force over these natural bodily urges.

The desires for food, sex, and comfort become the main purpose for survival and the only means to fulfilment in life. Relationships with others become the oppressive, jealous and disrespectful kind. With weak will power, we cannot help but be a slave to our own bodily urges, to fill these yearnings, which then corrupt our magnetism.
To develop this plane is to open the furthest limits of the mind to perform works that will be great and of lasting value. It is the cycle of apprenticeship in which success, without stress, depends on how we plan to use thought-power. In this respect, the dense conscious

mind must be supported within the fluidity of the intuitive creative part of the mind, of the corresponding fourth plane.

But this phase is best achieved when youth is in our favor, as the author of Ecclesiastes wrote describing the last days of dying man: "Remember now thy Creator in the days of thy youth, while the evil days come not, nor the years draw nigh, when thou shalt say, I have no pleasure in them". Such can only be achieved with knowledge founded upon Natural Laws at an early age. The mind that does this can only become stronger as one grows older and that which does not can only weaken.

A practical cast of mind stemming from *living* faith is bound to bring about a paradigm shift, *i.e.*, new transparencies. Individuals seeks purity of thoughts, flowing like the waves of water from which flows one's receptive clarity – the mind's natural state. Here, on the fourth plane of consciousness, thought-power is supported and nurtured by the fluid of the creative feminine principle. The result is impelled motion, which in joyousness of activity the seeker lives transcendental consciousness.

The fluid movement of this intuitive perceptive plane is what redefines and reopens the doors within oneself to a clearer perspective and a wiser application of the feminine in its most creative sense, with the understanding, however, that this dynamic comes whether the individual is in a masculine or feminine body. It is the principle that this plane is most concerned with, even though on the surface it might appear that one in a feminine body would have a deeper responsibility to such application. Here, it is the application itself and the approach, the belief systems attached to feminine and the ability to change such systems that is of the most importance and that comes no matter which body one inhabits.

Ascent to this plane of consciousness concerns one's readiness to seek. To open the doors of deep understanding of the feminine principle, the softer passive nature of the higher self. Opening up to the feminine mystique and the feminine nurturance and to recognise how it has been misused.

The same which applies to the woman's misuse of the masculine of the third plane remains so for man's misuse of the feminine on this plane, be it a woman's body or in his own creative mind. The man who represses his masculinity by engaging too much in the feminine energies of the mind allows his aggressiveness to be drawn off until he becomes effeminate. This is why we see men either born with the predisposition to feminine characteristics or heading in this direction. Men with broad hips and loose, or delicate muscle tone who are more comfortable in feminine activities.

A man bearing such a distortion can never rise to this plane of conscious activity, for naturally he lacks the higher substantiality of the primeval essence of feminine mystique and its nurturance. Neither can the one who misuses and abuses women, for he is without love from having suppressed his emotions and yield to the temperament of the brute. Both kinds are not masculine enough, *i.e.*, are weak and yielding. Yes, the male activates the birthing process but he cannot nurture it and give birth, be it to an idea, a child, or anything that pulses with life to come to full term. For what other reason does the woman bear womb and the man does not? The womb is but a symbol of the transformational nature of the feminine.

Only when the male is forced to recognise the feminine principle as that great help he need, and can never misuse if he wants to fulfil his task in life, then can he rise to this plane of spiritual self-consciousness. He will then relinquish his need for control and dominance, and swing in the fluid expression of the feminine - his compliment and creative source – be it with his mate or within his own consciousness. By so doing he also restores harmony with the rest of Creation in a more expansive way, in a blended nature of oneness of the heart. Consequently it keeps him from expressing only in an intellectual or abusive way, and nurtures the interconnectedness of himself.

He will find his sovereignty by the way he intuitively feels in his heart towards genuine womanhood. Whether his sovereign in all its queenly aspects be mother, mate, or just woman in general, it makes no difference. Finding "the bone of his bone and flesh of his flesh" he feels compelled to protect woman, because he feels himself *the stronger one* – in the physical sense, thus displays gentle consideration towards delicate feminine.

Having misused the feminine principle he must now "transpose the lights", that is, return the higher spiritual-creative feminine to above his cold, lifeless, calculating intellectual. It is on this plane life is transformed. Whereas on the previous plane we were our thoughts, in other words, our thoughts were reflected in our activities, on this plane we are now the observer of our thoughts. This movement challenges us to reflect deeply on our understanding of this creative-feminine aspect of self, to honestly see where we presently stand with it. Not with the thought-process of past self-assessment or validation, but to activate the lower "ego".

We could call it a cathartic approach wherein we observe every thought-volition, every pent-up emotion and false conviction within and shatter the destructive elements, clear out those outmoded belief systems. There can be no movement as long as we are not willing to look at the precepts, systems and boundaries we have already erected regarding the feminine and its fluid capacity to change and create.

It is said that only a few have attained the maturity for this conscious recognition in this epoch. A level of maturity should come seven years later from the previous stage – by the age of twenty eight. But whatever the cyclic or calendal age and whenever it happens, these are the human spirits who have made the invocation to have themselves freed from the flesh (matter) in time.

Movement spoken of here is not that which is thought or pondered – some small and intimate place within our soul or psyche. Not gained from self-actualisation seminars or workshops, psychotherapy, indoctrination or education, or some moral teachings we have studied either – although any of these factors can act as the catalyst. It is about knowledge gained only through experience on life's path. A movement wherein the intellect is so adequately developed that we experience it upon the body in the performance of work which becomes but a joyous play.

The joyous birth of any creative process has to be brought forth in some form to be clearly understood. The state of mind has to be of such that we are always ready to open and birth, if we are truly going to understand the heart of the feminine and its ability to nurture its creation whether that be the birth of a child, the birth of a country or nation, the birth of intimate relationship or the birth of the feminine within oneself.

Many a soul, however, after finding that they have for too long stubbornly followed a materialistic path, instead of humbly seeking spiritual guidance within, embark upon some of the most dangerous fly-by-night occult practices as they endeavor to exit their maze. All with the hope of developing themselves on this physic plane without consciously climbing the necessary intermediary step in an effort to at least shed this arrogance and conceit.

Hence it is said: Fools rush in where angels dare thread. Individuals so artificially developed find it difficult or impossible to discriminate between perception and illusion; between truth and deception; or between the thousands of ways thoughts work within this plane of creative formative substance. Any result can therefore prove decidedly dangerous for such ignorant ones; for it is a process which is a one-sided groping upwards over the intuitive perceptive bridge, instead of through deep reflective action. A bridge which can never be crossed other than by that conscious intercourse with mind and spirit, which alone brings about those experiences that give the higher power for psychic protection.

Such approaches remain mental and the consequences the same – the worst case scenario – madness. Even if one has a more or less natural psychic ability, like the finest swimmer, sooner or later he or she will eventually face limitations, because the waters are not their natural habitat. And a drowning person will catch at a straw. Only too late will one learn that they did not gain the consciousness experiencing that allowed them feel at home like a fish in water, which must always be on the alert for predators in its natural environment.

Likened to the swimmer, the development of this intermediary step is the actual connection on which any seeker who wants to move in this fluid creative process can hang as a counterbalance to their own psychic maturity. All that one would try to gain artificially is effortlessly given as to the swimmer with the right attitude.

After time, with much experience and renewed strength, like the fish in its natural terrain, this individual can then release the support, because they are one with the creative principle, they know the many-sided effects of this law. They know how to command the thought process to bring things to pass without endangering themselves and their environment.

This is therefore not the place for imagination, the product of the thought process. Imagination bears ethereal, but not spiritual, power. It is the joint working of intellect and feeling. Imagination consists of pictures we generate in the head, unrelated to the pictures formed by the spirit's perception. Our thoughts proceed from imagination in order to form the basis of our fantasy.

The pictures of imagination occur so rapidly that they seem like intuitive perception. They are, however, entirely different. Intuitive pictures are full of living power; pictures of the imagination are deceptive, the product of a far lesser power. Imagination only influence its creators, inflaming their enthusiasm, and never others. Not like intuitive power which creates, animates and emits radiations to fire and convince others. We cannot fake this development, for this plane mirrors the conscious brain. To do so would deceive oneself and others about spiritual matters.

Though we act on the intellectual plane and can front a facade, it is on this plane that all actions first take form. And if we fail to develop the capacity to observe ourselves, others so advanced can see through our pseudo-personality. Like all demands of truth, if we are sincere about transforming our beliefs and understanding, the intuitive mind can provide great glimpses into the possibilities of change, beyond time and space.

Only when we stand consciously in this movement do we prepare ourselves inwardly "to strive towards the ideal". Here the bandage of ignorance carefully and gradually begins to fall from our eyes now that our spirit is more clarified. The bandage which was placed in the character as a necessity that through such conscious experiencing, that at this clarified stage of our lives *only*, we may come to recognition of our own true nature – good or evil, likewise the nature of all things. And every part-step we take to this intermediary level must be deeply experienced in order to finally ensure the possibility of coming to this self-recognition, the basis for self-consciousness.

Ascent to this intuitive light-plane of pure perception, therefore, is what renders an individual a moral, responsible, and spiritual being; this ascent humanises, adorns and elevates one's nature; for it moulds the higher and nobler faculties. It begets aspirations after goodness, virtue, purity, and moral principles, and connect us with Nature's forces, angels and God. We learn to see ourselves and others as moral beings governed by Spiritual Laws contrasting previous selfish traits and passions. We internalise these Laws and values to develop the conscience.

What therefore underlines and brings about this feminine aspect of self, but love? The law through which we are able to recognise all wrong desires and actions and transmute them to this higher plane of self-conscious action. In many ways, this is a birthing plane and assists in the true birth within our lives in any and all ways that are aligned and appropriate with the manifestation of love. Love free from judgement, pain or punishment but manifested in our work as the progressive development of self. Only the true feminine knows love has no limits and exists within every form no matter its size, knowing or purpose.

This does not speak to that kind of love associated with our weaknesses. That which feeds others' selfishness, vanity, desire for ease, conceit, or sexual passions; which serves only to slide the one we think we love further along a downward path. It is love – the feminine principle – which demands that everything that is formed be kept and maintained in perpetual creative motion, with the strictest consistency. That which nurtures, supports and does only what benefits the other spiritually, which may call for severity, even cause pain if this is the only way one must be made to understand. We could call love quality control.

It is the love element of this plane that forms the bridge leading to the opening of the higher spiritualised self, from powerful radiations, to exercise dominion over our lower nature, *i.e.*, thought, feelings and emotions, of the three lower planes. Love is the means by which we can recognise our faults and weaknesses and advance spiritually. Together with the third plane is formed our metempericAL reality, consisting of thought and soul essence. One now easily adapts to the natural right and wrong of things, to the Natural Laws, the overall moral nature and constitution of things.

From higher spiritual planes the heart is now able to receive and radiate powerful currents through our words and actions. No longer reside those selfish propensities, but the desire to serve humanity. One is now more concerned with service based on human need than that of selfish motives. Creative endeavors are planned toward communities of interest. Nor can this love be directed to only one other, because only the whole of mankind can make the strings of such a matured soul, laid bare through purification, sound the chord of heavenly harmony. One bears this harmony within oneself, because all strings vibrate.

Living from this plane is to "live form the heart". That place where the attraction for earthly pleasures give way to the observance of high moral values – love, wisdom, logic. Because it is a "heart opening" plane, it facilitates deeper understanding of the nurturance of the heart, allowing us to give and receive form the heart and issuing out levels of pains when such fluidity (as giving and receiving) does not take place. But such suffering can only give way to our liberation when we adjust our behavior to the working of the creative principles.

We can therefore say that the reward of this conscious development is the gift of intuition (prophesy) – *living* faith; the "light within".

Here spiritual life truly begins. We now come to trust prophetic guidance; perception and feeling of the spiritual; interior perception of truth, what is best, what is about to transpire, *etc.*, that which forever warns. Here our conviction of a future is strengthened.

This self-conscious plane is therefore what gives us hope, the anticipation of success and happiness, if we look on *this* bright side. Dreams and ideals are built here. It magnifies, prospects, speculates, promises. It adapts our existence to God, and the pleasures and benefits experience in worship. A movement that makes one benevolent – the good Samaritan – self-sacrificing, neighborly.

Here truly is found the love for life; wit, pleasantness and laughter; intuitive perception of the ridiculous. One can only radiate this pure love energy, utter only wisdom and pure reason. Magnetically, those of like disposition and moral development are drawn together.

With perpetual striving, one can only be continually attracted upward to greater happiness and bliss through activity. And although conscious existence on this level also concerns our intellectual ability, it is not through the high development of the intellectual faculties that we ascend to higher spiritual planes, but due to a high moral development.

Here is where intellectuals, cognisant of their impotence, begin to persecute those who have shattered the walls of their limitations. We read and hear of this in the inquisition of the witches of the past and the court cases of alternative health practitioners of today. Interestingly, history's greatest atrocities were carried out by religious intellectuals, today by all those who seek to protect their intellectual prominence and financial gains.

As usual the State sided, and still sides, with the intellectuals. After thousands of years, they not only remain a danger to themselves but also to the world; for they believe they have the right to impose their limited convictions by law, erect obstacles for those of us who perceive reality otherwise. Anything they cannot validate scientifically with their dense brains, they call theory or quackery.

What intellectuals find difficult to understand is that knowledge lies only in the maturity of the spirit, in which concepts or forms change. Therefore there can be no hard and fast rule in that which is transitory, such as the intellect. Only the experience of the soul is real and eternal, always changing as we mature. In the Law of Continuous Motion, the creative feminine births newer and newer realities. Therefore only things which can be intellectualised belong to theory, never to true knowledge gained in experience. Knowledge which remains constant is not mobile, and, as such, cannot expand the mind.

Christ faced this denial and animosity by these so-called advanced ones who ceaselessly persecuted Him and worked for His earthly destruction. When they looked into their own depraved souls they saw that He was superior in His thinking and felt threatened. They sought always to discredit his credentials and social status.

Only at this fourth level of consciousness can understanding be gained to begin aligning body and spirit. The feminine intuitive perception originates in the mobility of the spirit and seeks union with the masculine active mind to change our genetic code, thus our attitude toward life. Developing this other part of the mind is the means to altering DNA, even slightly, in either direction while enscripting new ones. Good volition changes us for the better, no matter how inferior one's intelligence, or vile one's past; whereas evil thoughts corrupt our magnetism and lead to a pathetic life of crime, envy, hatred, lust and disease.

FIFTH PLANE – SELF-PERFECTING PLANE AND WILL POWER

This spiritual plane develops out of the former, representing the strict balance between "intellect and intuition", "feeling and emotion", "aggressive and passive" – the androgynous state. The state where the fiery intellect and the profusion of watery perception consummate to establish equanimity within the being. Or said otherwise: the passive love element of the feminine and the positive executing force of the masculine conceive to the Unified Self.

This is not about bisexuality, but a state wherein one's personal magnetism no longer emanates sexually but spiritually. The attraction to another is not for the sake of sexual desire and fulfilment but for spiritual ennoblement and fulfilment of our *life's work and purpose*. The human spirit ascends to its androgynous – unified – state, to its subconscious state before it descended into matter as unconscious spirit-germ in the quest for self-knowledge, only now it is self-conscious.

According to quantum theory this state is the Unified Field of all the Laws of Nature – Creative Intelligence. All aspects of the self are brought forward to be cleared and aligned with love as the key, the window, the door and the illumination. One aligns with self, others and the world in general. No longer is this enlightened individual able to access his or her reality from outmoded standards whether they come form self or others.

Hence the plane of the alpha and the omega of the spirit-seed in the World of Matter; the actual beginning (of the descent into the World of Dense Matter) and the end (of the traverse to gain *spirituality*). Unity becomes the objective of the seeker from here onwards, no more diversity. Reaching beyond self-made limitations the seeker perceives what once appeared as boundless diversity and separateness, connected parts through reciprocal effects. Now he or she is able to see that Creation itself which is a whole. It has no separate parts. The female and male are but one.

Only after the desperation to escape the constraints of life which kept the mind centered on everyday trivialities was one able to receive guidance toward this self-knowledge. The power is love. The seeker's life becomes a complete operation of love in action. And the supreme power of love continuously sweeps one upward with the impetuosity of a whirlwind to connect directly with God.

This plane of organised matter, we could say, is connected to the second, the third and fourth planes and serves as the bridge to the sixth, hence the bridge between spirit and matter. It was out of the unconscious Spiritual, came the urge to human development. A development which could only occur in the growth of the intellectual brain, as stimulated by the intuitive brain to attain conscious experience. Therefore if the mind is cultivated towards a spiritual goal and not the earthly passions – the once-manipulative sexual energy – it submits to the creative love of the feminine. A state of total surrender to the oneness of self and an outer expression of same.

Only in developing one's inner potentials can sexual energy flow upward from the lower planes as a result of the increasing activity. The ensuing control of the sensual organs prevents the dissipation of generative power given to us for creative pursuits. The materialistic quests and the insatiable appetite for food, sex, and comfort are subjugated – not suppressed – to this higher energy. No longer does the seeker waste time and money on perpetual motion, and other like futile contrivances. Instead perception and admiration of the beautiful, of poetry and fine music and literature develops, a sense of propriety, polish, love of Nature – personal neatness and finish.

The seeker is now ready to do what Jesus admonished: take up the cross and follow me. In other words, adapt oneself to the simplicity of the Laws of Creation, learn and understand them fully and make the best of their automatic effect, to escape the binding effects of karma in thoughts, words and actions.

The simplicity of the Divine Laws allows only great success where all the power is focused upon one point – the unified point, equanimity; where there is separation lies danger. The fact that that observing the Law of the Power of ever Simplification alone gives the victorious greatness which becomes effective in simplicity.

This Cross, however, must not be mistaken for the religious symbol of the Cross of Shame upon which Jesus was crucified – where the vertical masculine energy overpowers the horizontal feminine, but the equal armed Cross of Redemption which accords with Divine Will. The Cross wherein the horizontal and vertical beams of equal length and strength represents equal male and female. Though at first it appeared appeared separate to the neophyte, the aspirant experiences within that male and female are not definite species, but a manifestation of splitting which happened once in the Divine, and continued many times, finally, splitting in the Ethereal Plane (body). A body which still carries within itself the desire for a final union – the Unified Self.

It was to here that the flowery paths of pure sexual attraction between man and woman of the second plane was supposed to lead. That *union of perfect spiritual harmony* brought about by the desire to support each other's growth – in every word, thought and action and not mere sensual instinct and senseless desires. Such an earlier marriage was a journey to this new union, a second marriage, where man and woman can now truly "become one before God".

Here to be experienced for the first time is the bliss, the true pleasure of a union between the soul mates. No longer is pleasure sought from the procreative climax of coition, but from the joint union of creative climax in the sphere of activity, within the unified field of action of each other. The woman becomes the masculine in addition to herself, and the man vice-versa; and the intimate fusion and mutual exchange of energy serve to create a circuit of greater power for them. The union now becomes one of fulfilment, no sensual longing.

On this plane words become irrelevant. The bond of communion formed between like souls is such that the thought of the man resounds within the woman at the same moment; while the wishes of the woman is immediately carried out. One freely lives in the field of silence – transcendental – consciousness, even in the hustle and bustle of this modern world. A consciousness gained only in the sphere of activity geared towards uplifting humanity, not in reclusivity.

Soul mates, however, do not necessarily have to live together in marriage or be physically attracted to each other. As long as the spiritual goals of two people are complimentary, they need not be personally acquainted with each other. In fact, either could be involved in relationships with others which do not compliment their spiritual goal in life; mates who do not possess those qualities to fulfil a joint working of their *life's work and purpose*.

As each embark upon this journey in their separate worlds, though the path be steep and rocky, the inner experiencing of bliss will be to the same end. Nature becomes the complimentary husband and wife: in the perception and love of the grand, infinite, vast, illuminate, omnipotent, eternal and endless; of lofty summits, grand and stupendous towering mountains, rushing winds and storms, loud thunder and clapping lightning, majestic rivers, raging seas, burning volcanoes; to the cool caressing summer breeze, trickling streams and brooks, scintillating sunsets, delicate aromatic flowers in sunny meadows.

In the Laws of Creation, the perpetual desire to align body and spirit within the self through activity, forms a union which forces the completeness of the two split species within the self. If unmarried, there lives no burning desire to physically meet each another. For within both the separate souls are forged the Love of God ever more securely. The Love which was, is and forever remains the only support and stays throughout the tribulations and trials in life.

The lone aspirant sings only of the promised marriage to the Bridegroom, like the five wise virgins spoken of in the Parable Jesus gave. One who is not numbered among the five foolish virgins, of humanity. Those who are too lazy to exercise the necessary care and attention to tend to and keep their lamp in readiness; the lamp of discerning given them by the Creator. The correct application of the masculine and feminine principles established equanimity in the soul. Such workings alone allowed the seeker to draw oil from the depth of the soul, saturate the wick and burn a bright flame; the light of recognition, to be able to "see" the "Spirit of Truth", the Bridegroom, when He comes. The foolish ones are forced to remain behind with their rigid,outmoded beliefs, religious dogmas and creeds when the wakeful enter the Kingdom of Bliss.

And Nature supports this advancement. By the time this development occurs, in the most productive cycle for human creative achievements, one is no longer obsessed with amatory passions. Symbolically, it peaks at thirty five – the midway point of adulthood. It is said, however, that the female is most sexually active at this time, but only one who is consumed with sexual thoughts or nervous tension is unstable. If she is incensed within the fire of her life's work, she has neither time or energy for such self-consuming passions; even though gaining the equanimity she seeks can take the rest of her earth-life to develop.

By age forty-two cyclic ovarial function ends – menopause sets in. Estrogen, the hormone which controls female sexual development and child-bearing capacity, decreases and ends around the age of sixty; whereas the gonadotropic follicle stimulating hormones increases, *e.g.*, hair follicle, and levels off around age fifty to produce more sex hormones. The medium point of this rise and fall starts around age forty-eight, when ovaries begin to produce small amounts of androgens, the mainly testosterone hormone.

Androgens influence sexual differentiation and development, stimulating later development of the ovary. In the sexually undifferentiated embryo (androgynous state), it is the accepted theory that testosterone stimulates the development of the so-called Wolffian duct system, the presage of the male genital tract in mammals. Later, testosterone, along with gonadotrophins released by the pituitary gland, stimulates spermatogenesis. The Müllerian duct system, the presage of the female genital tract in the female embryo, is thought to have differentiated spontaneously without hormonal stimulus. After the female sex is well defined, estradiol, produced in the ovaries and the placenta, play a major role in the development and the functioning of the female reproductive tract.

This theory goes hand in hand with the Creation Story according to Genesis. Adam, speaks to the first set of androgynous or sexless human-spirits on earth, who, having to survive the turmoil in the rough elements in Nature developed the rougher, sterner intuitive perceptions. These were the first emotions to activate and dominate. This part was therefore called man. Accordingly, the delicate emotions of the spirit-seed had to be drawn off ethereally to form a separate species, and was later incarnated in gross material substance as woman.

This process splits the original spirit-seed into species, *i.e.*, smaller parts; that is, male and female, dependent upon each other. Each in its form represented the expression of the nature of the activity which it chose or desired.

This separation follows the Ethereal Law, in which everything takes on form; the delicate and passive manifest in female forms, the stern and the active in male forms. Here female and male have nothing to do with sex, but merely indicate the nature of their activity in Creation. The distinctive shape of the male from the female is but a coarsely constructed copy of this initial desire of the spirit-seed.

Hence a return to man's androgynous state (ethereally) sees a gradual increase of testosterone in the female's ovary as estrogen decreases. By mid-forties women's facial hair thickens and grows and their voices lower.

The designation of male and female by the procreative organ one bears is an animal classification, mistaken for the human spirit, in that the latter needed a material body for its development in the World of Matter. The procreative organs are for reproduction only, for uniting basic species, male and female, to bring about a renewal that accords with the Law of Creation – a renewal on the one hand which acts as a preserving agent (the nurturing feminine aspect) and on the other requires propagation (the compelling and energetic masculine aspect).

This plane can therefore be called the clearing house – the self-perfecting plane. One which does not deal with specific issues of masculinity or femininity but with the ability to balance the two. Here sexuality and its expression are brought into balance through opportunities which show themselves to release outmoded belief systems that are shrouded in guilt and misunderstanding so that healing can begin. Here all past hurts are felt and released so that the depths of trauma caused by them can be no more.

This is not to say that one suddenly comes out of one's personal closet. Rather a letting go of the trauma is possible to allow for a new understanding within self as to what is truly important in one's life. This experience is what it means to be "born again", born to a new life.

After this release, it is possible to see a physical change within the individual and in such a way that one can no longer identify easily the orientation of the person. This is not to say that there is not an expression of either the masculine or feminine body, rather a more fluid physical identity where one is not attached to maleness or femaleness, for both energies now work harmoniously within the same being. And since this clearing and alignment cannot sit on the outside where no one can see, it must manifest in the matured one's actions, where the individual brings into form a balanced awareness of one's experience and expression because in this androgynous state to execute will is to simultaneously form. The power of will determines the power of action.

At this higher reality, one manifests from deeper levels of the soul and connects to the outside world to significantly influence the sphere of action. We find here those individuals who have love and talents for the fine arts; for attaining whatever is beautiful and perfect; or improving it until it becomes so, and for any other mental activity involving creativity. In fact, all "blue prints" be they city and town plans, architecture, fashion design, painting, drawing, writing, *etc.*, are drawn from this plane of medium ethereal matter. The genetic coding for human life-form first developed from here, whether the soul today is developed or underdeveloped, spiritually advanced or primitive.

As the aspirants' intellect suffuse with spiritual-intuitive perception, the self-conscious individuals find waves of power issuing from their experiences in life which not only penetrate their thinking, but others'. In the same way that electrical current run through cable or that of invisible radio waves, even penetrating walls.

No longer can one be irresponsible and childish; for in the Laws of Creation whoever brings form to perfection must also take responsibility for the deed. Whether good or evil. Our volition, thinking and actions – everything – take on form in the creative process.

Keen observation develops to the point where one easily discovers discord or interruption in organised activity; for Nature supports all activity and gives the aspirant full comprehension of the working of its forces. Hence, in the strict logical sequence of happenings and at the proper timing, one is able to manifest form in *ordered* splendor, for the force of will is very strong. The aspirant is now able to command his or her thoughts. He or she calls on the faculty of thinking only when they want to bring into form what is thought of. Here humans truly are the "master of their own destiny".

One finds joy in activity, because to this creative human being everything flows. Creation offers everything of beauty it contains. Even beauty from the creative seedlings of a non-condensing, non-magnetic individual, that is, one who has fails to develop the gifts and abilities to this level. In this lies the meaning if the law: "from him that hath not, even that which he hath shall be taken away. Everything one needs, everything that brings joy and peace streams towards this individual as he or she dances in the joyfulness of the greatest happiness with the Natural Laws. In this heightened state of activity, true happiness is found, never before, no matter how hard we may try.

Only here can the human spirit truly serve the Creator through work that comes to life. Service to God gains a higher meaning. No longer is worship about religious ordinances and prayers, but that to honor God in the truest sense in *joyful activity* is to invest our talents in making use of everything Creation offers. The return is compound interest, in the greater perfecting of our work. Hence the principle: "To work is to pray".

This plane is the ultimate goal in the quest to self-consciousness – the ideal human being. It would have been easy to preoccupy oneself with one's own self-perfection, and that is alright, but our highest attainable goal is to make all effort to *uplift* existing things for the benefit of true humanity, not in the intellectual sense of increasing power and position, but towards ennobling them.

Here lies the total experience of the inner life of an individual, the height of personality ambition. The faculty of the so-called sixth sense is now fully developed for the emanation of spiritual energy. Accordingly, the adept experience the full opening of the "third eye", the organ of spiritual vision, which symbolises the perfect equipoise between the material and spiritual worlds. A fully developed right or intellectual brain represents insight, almost perfect spiritual vision; whereas the fully developed left intuitive brain, represents maturation of the lower, material aspects of the mind.

This makes it the plane of synthesis, of the abstract and the relative, of cause and effect. It is adapted to the first principles or laws. One so advanced knows all the Natural Laws for one lives them in daily life, by experiencing the absolute precision things gear into each other. They know of the unchangeability of the activity of these laws in their steady drive forward. In this steady observation their spirit kindles and is truly alert in their intuitive perception, thus become mobile in spirit.

Their spirit experiences pure bliss-consciousness which brings them in close communion with the Primordial Elemental Beings, otherwise called gods, and with angels. Their spirit moves with the radiance of solar velocity, represented by the two interlaced triangles, also known as the star of David. These are the true alchemist who has found the Philosopher's Stone, that is, the recognition of God in the Laws of Creation.

Since radiance of God (the upper triangle) cannot descend directly into matter, from here the human spirit (the lower inverted triangle) makes its way up in the rapture to the seventh plane, from where it originated. Such a person is truly vigilant. Like St. John in the Revelations he is at times brought to the seventh heaven to witness marvellous, yet unspeakable, things that shall come to pass.

Of this most ideal human being Jesus said: "Verily I say unto you, among them that are born of woman there has not one risen greater than John the Baptist". As the bearer of Divine Love in the purest form, of all his intuitive perceptions, thoughts and actions there was one-pointed love, loyalty and devotion to the service of God. Through his requisite exertion to fight "the sin" he became a fiery flame in his own enthusiasm.

The Book of Revelations refers to "the sin" as the beast with two horns. John is the man connected with the beast with two horns. He has the same number as the beast, in his inner equanimity. The number with the crushing power of the vibration of the Light – six hundred, three scores and six – 666. Cosmologically, the number 6 represents *might* – inner strength and equanimity.

This connection relates to the duality within the innermost self. To humans castrated in their own power of carnal desires by one-sidedly developing the intellectual (the beast), to pursue a life of sensuality and material acquisition. "The sin" is the intellectual war waged against the spirit, preventing it from, or leaving it no time to attain higher moral virtues. Having gained dominion, the intellect places itself on a throne above the spirit. Even more so today with people glorying in their conceit, arrogance and lust.

If we are to conquer the beast we must do as Jesus said, "watch and pray". We must forever be alert as to what emanates from our thoughts and perceptions, watch our selfish desires and motives. This alone gives true vigilance for self-conquest. At the same time we must pray not to fall into the snares and temptation of evil, by maintaining the connection to Luminous Spiritual Heights. Thus the verse of the Lord's Prayer: *Lead us not into temptation but deliver us from evil.*

Under the compulsion of this necessary resistance, the spirit finally glows and bursts into flames to consume every defect of character. In the end, having overcome all obstacles, the aspirant's flame becomes as consuming as the cherubim with flaming swords placed at the border of Paradise to guard its entrance, thus able to pass through to the seventh plane – Spiritual Heaven.

The Grail Legends speak of one with unequalled might, Parsifal, who would come and crush the serpent's head – the intellect – to restore the wasteland, that is, the exuding wound of the soul – which until now weakened the spiritual core. However, this coming is mistaken for a second incarnation of Jesus on earth.

The "Chalice" and the "Sword" are the two symbols of this battle. The chalice represents the feminine nurturing power and womanhood in general; whereas the sword represents the masculine executing power of the intellect and man.

The sword which inflicted the wound, that is, the intellectual domination brought about by today's patriarchal societies, will be wrestled away from the serpent by Parsifal – King of the Holy Grail. When in His hands, this same sword will become the weapon of healing in the new millennium – the final necessary knowledge void of religious dogmas and creeds; for it will place in deranged human brains that animating factor which leads it back from the path of spiritual death, to its spiritual origin.

The chalice is the life-giving, life-sustaining pure Love in the feminine. When again woman stands at her place, as ordained by the Creator, she will no longer waver in her beliefs nor be tempted by adversaries of the wrong principles, and "eat the apple." She will take the lead to spiritual heights and lead humanity accordingly.

When the two are again reunited, the feminine and masculine principles in Creation, *earthman* and *earthwoman*, the painful exuding wound of the human spirit will heal, bringing closure to the ongoing human wars and conflicts. Then will this world know harmony, peace and happiness as all begin to again strive to the ideal human being.
A soul like John's, however, rarely, if ever, blesses this planet. If one does, it is to carry out a special mission. A soul which in the fire of

volition joyfully treads these arduous steps to self-consciousness. One who possesses, even as a child, the moral integrity to sway and guide nations and peoples, and usually without formal education.

These are the seers, the sages and prophets, who know all human nature, having developed and cultivated the radiations or attributes of the collective human temperament. There is established harmony first within themselves and likewise towards all human beings, like notes of a melodious chorus. This is the Christ-consciousness individual. One who knows how to interpret and use circumstances as a guide to conduct and wisely prophesise the logical sequence of things to come.

SEVENTH PLANE – THE REALM OF SPIRITUAL SUBSTANTIALITY

This is Paradise. The plane (home) of the unconscious spiritual and to where the human spirit returns, but now as the self-conscious being. The human spirit fulfils the Law of Revolution, depicted by a serpent's head closing on its tail; for in this Law, like circulating blood in the physical body which issues from the heart and back, everything must return to its starting point.

This is the plane of selfless service to the Light of God. Although here rests the unconscious, on this plane is no blowing away or expiring of the spiritual ego. The only *dissolution* is the *cloaks* which covered the human spirit in its sojourn in the World of Matter in order to return here as a pure, unencumbered spiritual being, fully conscious of itself.

The ethereal bodies which previously became less dense and free of base desires had become so translucent and so light through joyous activity, enabling the shining core of the spiritual substance to break through ever more radiantly, until finally the last remnants of the ethereal body fell away as if consumed by flames at the gate Paradise. Then the human spirit, having attained a complete personality by reason of its perfect nature, now crosses the border, where seraphin stand guard.

Here is found no place of eternal rest. The urge is to swing purely and unconditionally in the Will of God, in this Eternal Realm of Joyous Activity, and wishing nothing else. To rest would be contrary to the creative Law of Movement which demands movement in every creature if it is to live.

There can be no more personal desires here either. In the lawful condition, a spiritual being with personal ambitions and goals cannot exist here, it would have to sink back to the sixth plane of self-conscious action.

This plane now forms the lowest bridge to higher realms of the unconscious spiritual to lower realms of material existence. It becomes the lowest plane of higher Spiritual Planes. It is a plane in which life is of two kinds. One is self-conscious human spirit yet unconscious of higher realities. The difference is what now gives the newly arrived spirit the impetus for further development. Any conscious development has its basis in the unconscious which, through association with the self-conscious human spirit's ego, is continually stimulated to attain further consciousness. In other words, in the conscious, which has the same qualities as unconscious, the urge for further development lies in the unconscious, which can only take place when consciousness increases.

In the first place, it was to come to ego-consciousness that the original spirit seed-germ descended into the World of Matter, since in its unconscious state it could only come to consciousness through experiencing. And this urge towards further development caused human spirit-seeds – the maturing ambitious germs of unconscious spirituality – to be ejected over the farthest boundary of this Sphere of Spiritual Substantiality – out of Paradise – into the World of Matter through the process of automatic release.

Having attained this logical development, the human spirit returns to Paradise, a self-conscious human spirit, yet, unconscious to higher planes of conscious spirit. From here it journeys upward to develop further consciousness, until it can ascend no further without losing self-consciousness, to serve forever in the *Eternal Kingdom of God.*

CHARACTER RECORD

Organic conditions which affect and indicate character is in seven degrees of power – very large, large, full, average, moderate, small, and very small – indicated by the seven numerals 7, 6, 5, 4, 3, 2, and 1.

Those organs and conditions marked 7, are sovereign in their influence over character and conduct, and, combining with those marked 6, direct and control the feelings and actions. Those marked 6, have a powerful and almost controlling influence, both singly, and especially in combination, and press smaller ones into service. Those marked 5, play subordinate parts, yet their influence is considerable, though more potential than evident. Those marked 4, have a medium influence, and mainly in combination with larger ones. Those marked 3, are below par, still more so in appearance; exert but a subordinate influence; and leave character defective in these respects. Those marked 2, are so deficient as easily to be perceived; leave their possessor weak and faulty in these respects, and should be cultivated; while those marked 1 render their possessor almost idiotic in these respects.

1. *The Practical Phrenologist* (Eugene W. Austin, N Y, p.2).
2. Article: *Humans & Ageing Process* (Harald Krebs).
3. *Physiological Psychology* (Dr. Norstand, Van, N Y).
4. The exchange of radiations between the dispensing animistic impulse from without and the upward movement of volition in the field of joyous activity.
5. See Part III.
6. Author of the Grail Message: *In the Light of Truth.*
7. Discussed in more detail in Part II
8. Female heads are half an inch to an inch smaller than that of the male.
9. The Practical Phrenologist: Size a Measure of Power, p.5.
10. ibid, pp 59-60.
11. *The Second Brain* (Harper Collins).
12. See Part II, The Vital Temperament.
13. *Isopathic/Homeopathic Materna Medica* (Semmlweis - Verlag, Germany, 1988, p. vi.).
14. See also discussion on the bodily temperaments in Part II.
15. Explained in Part II.
16. *Handbook of Personality Theory and Research* (Rand McNally & Company, Chicago, 1968, p.8).
17. Fizlol. Zhurnal, (1954, Vol. 40 (5), p.618).
18. *The Mental Aspect in the Etiology and Treatment of Pulmonary Tuberculosis* (International Clinics, 1933, Vol III, pp 149-74), and French, Thomas & Alexander Franz, *Psychogenic Factors in Bronchial Asthma* Report I, *Psycho-somatic Medicine*, Monograph iv, 1941, p. 236.
19. A tendency of the body to secrete mucous and form tissues.
20. The balanced and integrated functioning of mind and body.
21. Temperament, Character and Personality (Simonov, P.V., & Ershov, P.M., 1984, p.7).
22. Nutritional Enzyme Support system (NESS) manual, (Riverside, MO 64150).
23. The 2nd person singular is used here because it is established, spiritually, that a child does not become a person, that is, responsible for its action until the spirit awakens at puberty.
24. Back to the androgynous state.

The Grail Message of Abd-ru-shin (1971), In the Light of Truth, Stiftung Gralsbotschaft Publishing Co., Stuttgart.

Fowler, O. S. (1869) *The Practical Phrenologist*, Eugene W. Austin, NY

Vollman, H. (1985) *A Gate Opens*, Stiftung Gralsbotschaft Publishing Co., Stuttgart.

Keirsey, David; Bates, Marilyn (1984), *Please Understand Me*, Gnosology Books Ltd.

Simonov P.V.; Ershov, P. M (1991), *Temperament, Character and Personality*, Gordon and Breach Science Publishers S.A.

Davies, John D (1955), *Phrenology, Fad and Science*, Yale University Press.

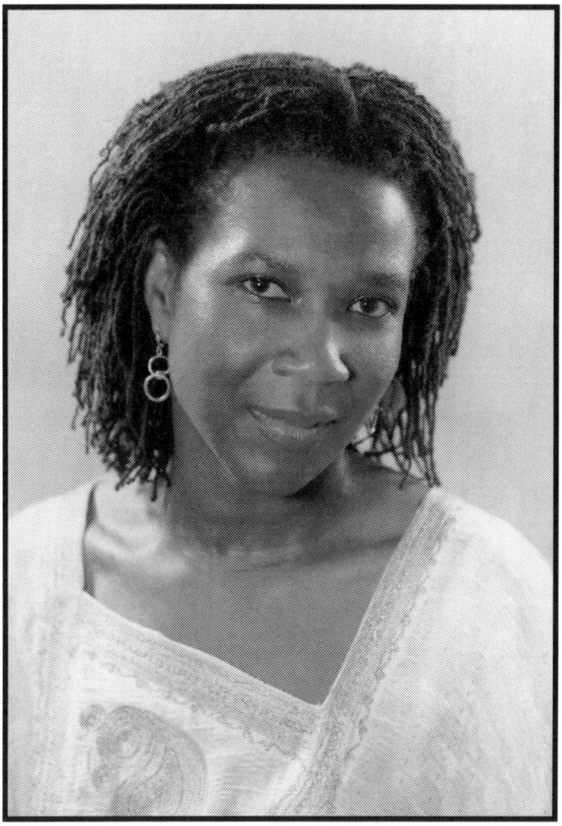

Monica Palmer (Tsheba) was born in Jamaica, West Indies, in 1959. After migrating to Canada in 1982, she entered the field of natural medicine and is today a renowned therapist and ontological coach in Toronto. For over 10 years she has helped many nutritionally, not only to obviate stress, sickness or its genetic disposition, but also establish and maintain equanimity between body and spirit, through changing their way of thinking and moderating their excesses.